Keto Diet Meal Plan For Beginners

14-Day Diet Meal Plan for

Weight Loss and Healthy Living

BY STACY OLIVER

Table of Contents

Introduction

You are well on the way to a successful weight loss plan using the ketogenic techniques described in the *Keto Diet Meal Plan for Beginners: 14-Day Keto Diet Meal Plan for Weight Loss and Healthy Living*. The following chapters will discuss how to follow the plan and the ways it will most benefit your health. You will never feel deprived using the recipes as described in this book.

As you surround yourself with all of the healthier food choices, including an array of fruits and vegetables, you will discover how simple it is to enjoy the menus you love. You may need to make a few lifestyle changes to drop the pounds, but with the structured keto diet plan, the journey is much healthier in comparison to some of the 'fad' diets circulating around the Internet.

This diet plan has been around since the Middle Ages and is known for its ability to help with those afflicted with epilepsy. Epilepsy has puzzled many of the great thinkers of the last 4,000 years. The Greeks once referred to it as 'the sacred disease,' believing the gods gave it to humans. Hippocrates, an ancient Greek physician and 'the father of medicine,' disagreed with this notion. He wrote that the disease "has a natural cause, and it's supposed divine origin is due to men's inexperience and to their wonder at its peculiar character."

Attempts to characterize the condition were not accepted, and treatments were just as rare. The primary method for dealing with epileptic episodes was to run and hide before the seizures began. The term epilepsy itself derives from a Greek word meaning 'possessed.'

As time moved on, fasting was theorized by Bernard McFadden/Bernarr Macfadden as a means for restoring your health. One of his students introduced a treatment for epilepsy using the same plan. In 1912, it was reported by the *New York Medical Journal* that fasting is a successful method to treat epileptic patients, followed by a sugar and starch-free diet.

Just a few years later, in 1921, Rollin Woodyatt, an endocrinologist, noted the ketone bodies (3 water-soluble compounds; β-hydroxybutyrate, acetone, and acetoacetate) were produced by the liver because of a diet low in carbohydrates and rich in fat. In the same year, Dr. Russell Wilder who worked for the Mayo Clinic became well known when he formulated the ketogenic format that was then used as part of the epilepsy therapy treatment plan. He had a massive interest in the program because he also suffered from epilepsy. The idea also became known for its other effects that helped in weight loss and many other ailments.

The two doctors, in their quest for a treatment, notice a remarkable phenomenon when they placed their epileptic subjects on a restricted vegetarian diet or outright fasting. The frequency and severity of these epileptic seizures drastically reduced.

Now, you will learn of more benefits the diet plan has to offer, so you will fully understand whether the program will work for you. There are plenty of books on this subject in the market, thanks again for choosing this one! Every effort was made to ensure it is full of as much useful information as possible. Enjoy each chapter and plan ahead to know, you will always be prepared and never hungry once you have the plan in motion for a few weeks or months. You will get there!

CHAPTER 1

Tips to Achieve Ketosis & Benefits of the Ketogenic Plan

The Best Advice: Keep It Simple: Each of the recipes provided have been calculated for you. You have two weeks of menu plans before you are on your own. Take time out of your busy schedule to plan a week of basic meals. As long as you remain within your personal guidelines for weight loss; the recipes will help you reach them and beyond.

It is essential to go at your own pace and not become overwhelmed. Stop and take a deep breath. Let your body tell you what it needs. Everyone is different, and this point cannot be stressed enough since even if you have the same weight, you can have unique Basal Metabolic Rate or BMR. Just remember, this is a lifestyle change, not a race.

No matter what reasons you have for choosing the keto plan, you may hear others state that the program is not good for you. The problem being is that they do not understand the process of how the plan uses high-fats and low carbs in unison to keep you full and remain healthy. The human body needs lean fats that can be broken down to prevent long-term health issues.

You are essentially trying to recharge your metabolism. The process will begin as a detoxification process that may cause you to suffer from headaches or nausea. This is all a part of the process as the body fights a natural way to adjust for the lack of carbohydrates and 'junk foods' you have been consuming in the past. It should subside after a week or so. (More on this later.)

Dairy & Your Diet

Before beginning the keto way of life, you need to understand dairy and dairy products are an essential part of the ketogenic methods. If you are lactose intolerant; maybe the plan isn't for you. However, if you do, keep it at about 4 ounces each day.

Set Your Body's Building Blocks

In many cases, you are currently burning glucose as your 'fuel' source that, in turn, changes your food into energy. The remainder of the glucose develops into fat and is stored in your body to be consumed later.

The keto diet will set up your body to deplete the stored glucose. Once that is accomplished, your body will focus on diminishing the stored fat we have saved as fuel. The new technique will begin with 75% fats, 5% for carbs, and 20% for protein daily. Many people don't understand that counting calories do not matter at this point. It is just used as a baseline.

Two elements that occur when your body doesn't need the glucose:

- **The Stage of Lipogenesis:** If there is a sufficient supply of glycogen in your liver and muscles, any excess is converted to fat and stored.

- **The Stage of Glycogenesis:** The excess of glucose converts to glycogen and is stored in the muscles and liver. Research indicates that only about half of your energy used daily can be saved as glycogen.

Your body will have no more food (similar to when you are sleeping) making your body burn the fat to create ketones. Once the ketones break down the fats, which generate fatty acids, they will burn-off in the liver through beta-oxidation.

Thus, when you no longer have a supply of glycogen or glucose, ketosis begins and will use the consumed/stored fat as energy.

The Internet provides you with a keto calculator at "keto-calculator.ankerl.com." You can check your levels when you want to know what essentials your body needs during the course of your dieting plan or afterward. You will document your personal information such as height and weight. The calculator will provide you with the essential math.

When the glycerol and fatty acid molecules are released, the ketogenesis process begins, and acetoacetate is produced. The Acetoacetate is converted to two types of ketone units:

- **Acetone:** This is mostly excreted as waste but can also be metabolized into glucose. This is the reason individuals on a ketogenic diet will experience a distinctive smelly breath.
- **Beta-hydroxybutyrate or BHB:** Your muscles will convert the acetoacetate into BHB which will fuel your brain after you have been on the keto diet for a short time.

Choose the Right Plan To Enter Ketosis

An essential element of the ketogenic diet is that it is very flexible. As stated, you are different from everyone else. You have several options of using the ketogenic plan to your best benefits including:

- *Provision # 1*: You can choose from the standard ketogenic diet (SKD) which consists of high fat, moderate protein, and is extremely low in carbs.

- *Provision # 2*: The cyclical ketogenic diet or CKD is created with 5-keto days trailed by two high-carb days.

- *Provision # 3*: The high-protein ketogenic diet is very similar to the standard keto plan (described above) in all aspects; except that it has more protein.

- *Provision # 4*: The targeted keto diet, which is also called TKD, will provide you with a plan to add carbs to the diet during the times when you are working out.

These are the basic plans to get you started in the right direction. For beginners, you will probably use the first option. You may be asking what these macronutrients are, right?

Macronutrients

The macronutrients are building blocks of food consisting of protein, fat, and carbs. For a regular American diet, you may have a diet composed of 16% protein, 34% of calories from fat, and approximately 50% of the calories from carbs. As mentioned earlier, the ketogenic technique mixes it up with about 25% protein, 70% fat, and 5% from carbohydrates.

Everyone's totals are different since your percentages are calculated according to your weight, age, gender, body fat percentage, and activity levels. You can go online and type in *Ruled Me* or other sites and use the keywords *'keto macro calculator'* to locate the scale guideline. Just type in your information, and it will provide you with your macro limits.

Track the macros either by hand or by the use of a particular app such as *SparkPeople* or *MyFitnessPal*. This is the most accurate way to ensure you are remaining in ketosis and have no danger of over-eating. Use any method that works for you. Once you have the numbers, you are ready to go!

How Protein Balances Weight Loss

Protein is essential for your weight loss program and is a necessary part of the ketogenic diet. These are some of the most important reasons why you must include a balanced supply of protein in your diet:

Muscle Repair and Growth: Protein should be increased on days when you are more active. It is essential to have a plan for what your meals will consist of with a balance of carbs, proteins, and calories. The balance is what you are attempting to achieve with a focused plan such as the keto diet.

Protein Saves Your Calories: Protein slows down your digestion process making you feel more satisfied with the foods you eat. During the first cycle of your diet plan; it is imperative that you feel full, so there is no temptation to cheat on the strategy.

Protein is a Fat Burner: Science has proven your body cannot use and burn your fat as energy sources unless you have help from either carbs or protein. The balance of protein must be maintained to preserve your calorie-burning lean muscles.

How to Balance the Carbs

Research has indicated the methods used in the ketogenic diet plan are successful in approximately 90% of cases. The main chore you have (other than the workout) is keeping accurate records of your carbohydrate intake. Since there's no set rule, you'll want to be sure you are providing your body with the right amounts of food to keep your diet balanced for the state of ketosis.

You will be gradually working your way through the plan based on these food options. You should also consume a minimal intake of carbs, an abundance of fresh vegetables, and two to three pieces of fruit daily.

Your Daily Intake of 0-20 Grams of Net Carbs: You will discover most of the foods in this meal plan are dedicated to 20 or just above 20 grams daily.

Your Daily Intake Of 20-50 Grams: If you are obese, have diabetes, or metabolically deranged, this is the plan for you. If you are consuming less than the 50 grams daily; your body will achieve a ketosis status which will supply the ketone bodies. Just remember, to lose the weight according to the ketogenic technique, you will need to count those carbs.

Your Moderate Intake Amounting To 100-150 Grams Daily: If you are lean and maintain an active lifestyle, you may be trying to manage your weight.

Take the Right Steps to Ketosis

Even though ketosis will become a way of life, you may be a little confused on how it all works together. These are some of the ways to get the plan flowing so you can be in ketosis quickly:

Step 1: Consume Protein Daily

You must supply your liver with amino acids that can be used for making new glucose (gluconeogenesis). Your liver produces the glucose for the cells and organs in your body that cannot use ketones as fuel. This includes portions of the brain, kidneys and red blood cells. Protein also maintains muscle mass when the carb intake is lowered, especially during a weight loss program.

Step 2: Healthy Fat Intake Is Essential to Ketosis

Forget the old sayings that it has too much fat. Consuming plenty of healthy fats can help boost your ketone levels. The lowered carbohydrate intake teams up with the high fats to produce ketosis. If you are using the ketogenic diet for weight loss, you can also achieve 60-80% of your calories from fat. Note, the traditional diet plan for epilepsy is higher with 85-90% of the calories from fat.

It is essential to use high-quality food sources since you are consuming such a large percentage of your diet from fat intake. Consider using these good fats for your cooking needs; butter, coconut oil, avocado oil, and lard. You will soon discover how many high-fat foods are low in carbs, but you still need to count them to prevent losing the ketosis state. In general, you should consume a minimum of 60% of calories from fat to boost the ketone levels. Choose from both animal and plant sources.

Step 3: Maintain Ketosis, Add Coconut Oil

Coconut oil is also used as one of the best ways to improve ketone levels in people with nervous system disorders, such as those with Alzheimer's disease. The oil contains medium-chain triglycerides (MCTs) which speed up the ketosis process. Unlike many other fats, the MCTs are absorbed rapidly and go directly to the liver where they are used for immediate energy – resulting in conversion to ketones.

The oil contains four types of these fats, 50% of which comes from lauric acid. Research has indicated the higher percentage may produce sustained ketosis levels because it is metabolized more gradual than other MCTs. Add coconut oil slowly to your diet because it can cause some diarrhea and stomach cramping until you adjust. Begin with one teaspoon daily, and work it up to two to three tablespoons over the span of a week.

Step 4: Maintain a Low-Carb Diet Plan

One extremely vital element in achieving ketosis is a low-carbohydrate diet. Your cells usually use the sugar/glucose as the primary fuel source, but most of your cells can also use other sources for fuel such as fatty acids as well as ketones.

When the carb intake is lowered, the levels of the insulin hormone decline which allows the fatty acids to be released from fat storage in your body.

The formula to limit their intake of net carbs is this: Total carbs (-) fiber = 20 grams daily. However, some can remain in ketosis while eating twice that amount. If you can restrict your intake to 20 or fewer grams for the first two weeks, you should be well on the way to ketosis. At that time, you can relax and maintain the ketosis state.

Step 5: Test the Ketone Levels & Adjust the Diet Plan

Maintaining ketosis is an individual process. You must be sure you are achieving your goals. The levels of acetone, acetoacetate, and beta-hydroxybutyrate can be measured in your breath, urine, and blood. You can purchase a Ketonix meter to measure your breath. You breathe into the meter, and a color will flash to show your levels of ketosis.

You can also measure the ketones with a blood ketone meter which works similar to a glucose meter. Merely, add a small drop of blood on a testing strip and insert the tab into the meter. It will indicate the amount of beta-hydroxybutyrate in your bloodstream. This process has been researched as a valid indicator of the current ketosis levels. However, the strips are expensive.

The final choice is testing your urine for acetoacetates. The strip is dipped into the urine which will change the color of the strip. The various shades of purple and pink indicate the levels of the ketones. The darker the color on the testing strip; the higher the level of ketones. The significant benefit is they are inexpensive. The most effective time to test is early morning after a ketogenic diet dinner the evening before testing.

You should attempt to use one or more of these methods to indicate whether you need to adjust your intake of foods to remain in ketosis. However, you should be showing physical signs as well.

Your Eating Habits Balanced With Exercise

Exercise is a significant element to the success of the ketogenic diet plan.

Cortisol is a hormone which is released from your adrenal gland in response to chemical signs or other stress signals. The release of cortisol in long workouts, such as jogging, and the adverse effects of the release of high doses of cortisol for weight loss are essential elements in your successful program. The hormone creates the fight-or-flight reaction as a result of the additional activity/stress during your workout.

You should consider exercising 30-60 minutes daily as an integral part of healthy living choices. Regular physical activity benefits your strength, mood, and balance. If you have been living a more sedentary lifestyle, it's vital for you to speak with your doctor about a safe exercise regimen. Make sure you start off slow. Progressively 'pick up the pace' and regularity of your workouts.

Bump it up a notch and try intermittent fasting using your ketogenic techniques and recipes. Your metabolic rate is increased with short-term fasting because of the hormonal changes ranging in categories of 3.6% to 14%. Studies have established weight loss after three to twenty-four weeks on the intermittent fasting program to maintain losses of 3.0 to 8.0%. In comparison to other studies on weight loss, these are high percentages that cannot be ignored.

In the same studies, many of the individuals lost 4.0 to 7.0% of his/her waist circumference. This is an indication of how the harmful buildup of belly fat can cause disease and other issues around your organs. You have to consider these results are from eating fewer overall calories, and not binging during the days off. You have to maintain a sensible eating program.

While the core ideas behind the various forms of intermittent fasting are all the same, there are quite a few different ways to go about it. Your best bet is to try a few and see which one your body naturally responds to the easiest.

Intermittent Fasting: Option # 1, Eat-Stop-Eat

This form of fasting can be considered the most beneficial to those who are already eating healthy but want to give their weight loss an extra boost. On this type of program, you don't eat anything one or two days a week. During this period, you should only consume foods that have zero calories including black coffee (a splash of cream is fine), water, diet soda, and sugar-free gum.

When you are finished fasting, it is important not to overeat more than average and always to avoid binging for extended periods of fast/binge cycles can cause severe damage to your body. As always, it is important to practice moderation and self-control to get the most out of the fasting cycle.

This fast cycle works on the assumption that in to lose a pound of weight a week, all you need to do is give up 3,500 calories. So, it might be best to get it out of the way in two quick bursts rather than fasting for a portion of every single day. This fasting plan emphasizes resistance weight training for maximum benefits.

Going a full day without eating can be difficult for some people at first, but it is perfectly acceptable to work up to a full day of fasting by holding out as long as possible and increasing that amount of time with practice. An excellent way to start is by choosing days that you know don't have any prior food commitments. Beginning a fasting program on a day when you know you have a lunch meeting is just a depraved idea.

When first starting this fast cycle, fatigue, headaches, feelings of anger or anxiousness are all common side-effects and should be considered a good stopping point for your current fast. These side-effects will diminish as your body adjusts to the new cycle.

After going a full day without any calories, it will be natural to have the desire to binge during your first meal. You must use your self-control to fight these urges since not only is binging bad for you; it can quickly undo all of your hard work from the previous 24 hours. Practice self-discipline and make your fasting worth the effort.

Intermittent Fasting: Option #2, 16:8 Method

This method involves fasting for 16 hours for men, or 14 hours for women, before allowing a reasonable number of calories for the remaining 8 to 10 hours. During this period, (once again) you should only consume items that have zero calories including black coffee (a splash of cream is okay), water, diet soda, and sugar-free gum. The easiest way to attempt this schedule is to stop eating after dinner in the evening and wait 14 or 16 hours from there. This means skipping breakfast and picking things up in the early afternoon.

Again, the specifics of when you fast are not nearly as important as ensuring that you fast for the same period as regularly as possible. If you vary your fasting period too much, it can lead to an erratic change in your hormones, which among other things; make it much more difficult for your body to shed any excess weight. If you find yourself without the time required to eat a proper meal to break the fast with a regular meal - you must eat something to keep your body on the correct cycle.

If you are exercising, as well as intermittently fasting, it is critical to ensure that you are eating more carbohydrates than fats while you are working out, while on days you are not exercising the opposite is true. It is vital to ensure - every day you keep your protein intake at a steady level. As always, stay away from processed foods whenever possible.

One of the most significant benefits of this type of fasting is that it's incredibly flexible so that it will work for a variety of schedules. Most people find it helpful to either eat two large meals during the 8 or 10-hour period feeding period or split that time into three smaller meals as that is the way most people are already programmed.

On days you are exercising as well as fasting, it is essential to try and always break your fast with a mix of protein, vegetables, and fruit. If you generally go to the gym directly after you have broken your fast, it is important to include enough carbohydrates to give your muscles the energy they need to get the most out of your workout.

If you are planning to exercise, it is usually best to start the early afternoon healthy with a medium calorie meal. Then, just exercise within three hours prior to consuming a more substantial meal soon afterward. In this meal, it is essential to add a significant portion of complex carbohydrates. You can even have a little dessert as long as it is in moderation. Remember, fasting is different than dieting.

On days you do not plan on exercising, it is important to adjust your caloric intake appropriately. Start by limiting your carbohydrate intake, and instead focus on eating lots of protein, dark green, leafy vegetables and fruit in moderation. Unlike on days you are exercising, the first meal you eat on rest days should be your largest regarding caloric intake with this one meal counting for about 40 percent of your daily total.

Remember, during this meal, you should be taking in more protein than anything else. For your final meal during the 'rest' days; it's essential to include a protein source that will take lots of time to digest which in turn means it will keep you full for more of your fast the following morning. It also provides the body with enough stored amino acids to prevent it from breaking down muscle during the fast.

Intermittent Fasting: Option #3, Alternate Day Diet

This form of intermittent fasting actually means you never have to go long without food, if you so choose. Every other day you eat as usual, and on the off-days, you merely consume one-fifth of the calories you take in on the regular days. The average daily caloric consumption is between 2,000 and 2,500 calories which mean that the regular off-day varies between 400 and 500 calories. If you enjoy exercising every day, then this form of intermittent fasting may not be for you since you will have to limit your workouts on off-days severely.

When you first start this form of intermittent fasting, the easiest way to make it through the low-calorie days is by trying any one of a variety of protein shakes. It is important to work back to 'real' natural foods on these days because they will always be healthier than the shakes.

This form of intermittent fasting is all about losing weight. Those who try it tend to average between two and three pounds lost per week. If you attempt the Alternate Day Diet, it is imperative to eat regularly on your full-calorie days. Binging will not only negate any progress you have made, but it can also cause severe damage to your body if continued over time.

Individuals Who Reap Benefit using the Keto Plan

Specific groups of people benefit hugely from the techniques used including those who are at risk for some forms of cancer, diabetes, Alzheimer's disease, and many more. These are some of those benefits described in depth:

Increased Energy: As your body breaks down the fats instead of carbs. Think of the balance using the energy content of nutrients.

Successful Weight Loss: As you reduce the carbohydrate intake in your body, you will also be increasing the fats included in your keto diet. The multitude of fats, fibrous veggies, and satiating nutrients provided in the new diet. The 'full' factor is also a significant benefit to the ketogenic plan. You will not be hungry if you follow the program.

Insomnia: Experiencing a lack of sleep is also a typical side effect. Vitamin supplements can sometimes remedy the problem that can be caused by a lowered insulin and serotonin level. For a quick fix; try 1/2 of a tablespoon of fruit spread and a square of chocolate.

Lowered Triglycerides: Another natural process is involved as your body converts the excess of calories into triglycerides which are stored in the body's fat cells. It is an automatic response since an increased intake of unsaturated fats will automatically lead to a reduction in your blood triglyceride levels. Many experts suggest fatty fish consumption at least once or twice weekly to help reduce the risk of stroke.

More Control of Blood Sugar Levels & Insulin Usage: The increased carbohydrate intake is broken down into glucose - a type of blood sugar. High levels of blood sugar/glucose are toxic to your body. As a result, your body starts producing insulin which elevates your blood sugar levels. With the ketogenic diet, you are cutting out the carbs. Therefore, you can lower your insulin levels and blood sugar.

Polycystic Ovary Syndrome (PCOS): This is the utmost endocrine disorder affecting young women of child-bearing years and is also associated with insulin resistance, obesity, and hyperinsulinemia. A 6-month study concluded a significant improvement in weight and fasting women over a 24-week period. The group limited carb intake to 20 grams daily for the 24 weeks.

Boosted Cognitive Performance: Due to the reduction of glucose; your brain will begin to use ketones as fuel. As a result, the level of toxins will decrease. You will increase your productivity and concentration will improve.

Gum Disease and Tooth Decay: The pH balance in your mouth is influenced by sugar intake. Your gum issues could subside after about three months on a keto diet plan. You will be consuming healthier foods.

Acne: By eating fewer processed foods and less sugar; your insulin levels will be lowered, and the acne should improve.

Possible Ill-Effects of the Ketogenic Techniques

Your body will be making many changes during the first few weeks. You may have some of the issues as described in this segment. Don't stress about the problems, because they will be short-lived once your body reaches ketosis.

You may begin to feel 'fluttery' because of dehydration or because of an insufficient intake of salt. Try to adjust, but if you don't feel better quickly, you should seek emergency care.

You may experience what is called the 'keto flu' or 'induction flu' which involves lowered mental functions and energy. You may suffer from sleeping issues, bouts of nausea, increased hunger, or other possible digestive worries. Several days into the plan should remedy these effects. If not, add 1/2 of a teaspoon of salt to a glass of water and drink it to help with the side effects. You may need to do this once a day in the first week, and it could take about 15 to 20 minutes before it helps. It will go away!

As your body reaches ketosis, you may experience a fruity smell similar to nail polish. It is not unusual because the aroma is acetone which is a ketone element. Your body may also have an unpleasant odor as your diet changes. Just remember, to maintain good oral health and use remedies to improve your breath. Use sugar-free gum as a last resort.

Leg cramps may be an issue as you begin ketosis. The loss of magnesium (a mineral) can be a demon and create a bit of pain with the onset of the keto diet plan changes. With the loss of the minerals during urination, you could experience bouts of cramps in your legs.

Your urine will also react to the high acetone levels - which is yet another indication of your ketosis state. It is just your body adjusting to the new source of vitamins, minerals, and other nutrients.

It is possible for you to experience digestive issues. You have made an enormous change in your diet overnight; it's expected you may have problems including constipation or diarrhea when you first start the keto diet. Each person is different, and it will depend on what foods you have chosen to eat to increase your fiber intake using various vegetables.

You may experience issues because your fiber intake may be too high in comparison to your previous diet. Try reducing certain 'new' foods until the transitional phase of keto is concluded. It should clear up with time. You may be lacking beneficial bacteria. Try consuming fermented foods to increase your probiotics and aid digestion. You can benefit from b, vitamins, omega 3 fatty acids, and beneficial enzymes as well.

Similar to other diets, it will take consistency and total dedication to be successful with your new way of life. The issues described should subside after you have been on the plan for several weeks. Everyone is different, so your timing may be a bit different from other dieters.

Know What Foods You'll Avoid on the Ketogenic Diet

After you better understand your new diet technique, you will want to purge your pantry, refrigerator, and freezer of items that will not be on your menu in the future. You have so many choices to enjoy for your ketogenic diet plan, but you will discover quickly which ones need to be left out of your menu plan. These are a few of the demons you need to be aware of in the early stages of your new dieting experience. They include the following:

Avoid Unhealthy Fats: Limit use of the following fats. Occasionally, will be acceptable since your diet plan is flexible, just not every day.

- *Processed Trans Fats*: Avoid fast foods, processed foods, margarine, and commercially prepared baked goods.
- *Processed Polyunsaturated Fats*: Avoid these oils: Sunflower, peanut, grapeseed, sesame, corn, canola, and soybean.

Sugary Foods: Leave the usual 'junk foods' alone including soda, many fruit juices, cake, ice cream, and candy.

According to a favorite source, here are some processed snacks to avoid while on a ketogenic diet. Some are surprising because they were deemed for years as a healthy snack. Do you recognize any of them?

- Cereal Bars
- Rice cakes
- Flavored Nuts
- Popcorn
- Potato Chips
- Pretzels
- Protein Bars
- Crackers

If you see carrageenan on the label, it is best to leave it on the shelf. It is an extract from red seaweed which is also known as Irish Moss. It has been used traditionally for hundreds of years. It is found in cottage cheese, non-dairy milk, pudding, jelly, and ice cream - among others.

Don't feel too guilty if you crave all of those processed foods. It's normal. As a rule of thumb, look for labels with the least amount of ingredients. Usually, the ones that provide the most nutrition are listed in those 'short' lists.

Foods to Enjoy Occasionally

- You may use these occasionally, but you need to realize that they can add extra carbs to your recipes. You will also notice some of them listed in recipes. You just need to be aware that if eaten in large quantities is not focusing on your goals of ketosis.

- *Beans and Legumes:* This group to avoid includes peas, lentils, kidney beans, and chickpeas. If you use them, be sure to count the carbs, protein, and fat content.

- *Agave Nectar:* One teaspoon has 5 grams of carbs versus 4 grams of table sugar.

- *Nut or Seed-Based Products:* These items should be monitored since they contain high inflammatory Omega-6s which include corn oil, sunflower oil, almonds, pine nuts or walnuts.

- *Cashews and Pistachios:* The high carb content should be monitored for these yummy nuts.

- *Fruits:* Raspberries, blueberries, and cranberries contain high sugar content. In small portions, you can enjoy some strawberries, apples, or pears.

- *Diet Soda:* Artificial sweeteners can cause you to go out of ketosis if you consume large amounts of diet drinks. Therefore, you have to use it in moderation. Research has shown a link between artificial sweeteners and sugar cravings, making it more challenging to curb those types of drink.

- *Alcohol Beverages:* Limit the intake of your alcoholic **drinks to include:**

    a. Cocktails

    b. Flavored liquor

    c. Beer

    d. Dry Wine

    e. Mixers: Soda, Juice, or Syrup

The experts have discovered these may be acceptable occasionally:

    a. Vodka: Check the carb content since it is usually produced (grain-based) from rye, potatoes, and wheat.

    b. Rum: Choose the ones with zero carbs or sugar.

    c. Tequila: The agave plant is the source of tequila.

    d. Whiskey, Barley, corn, rye, and wheat are the grains used which have zero carbs or sugar.

Notice for Consumers: This doesn't promote you drinking alcohol, it still needs to be consumed in small amounts to prevent any health issues.

Enjoy Your Healthier Food Choices

Whenever possible, choose free-range or organic food items. For example, it's advisable to choose raw and organic milk products. You can also use full-fat products over low-fat or fat-free products.

Even with a hectic lifestyle, it is vital for you to have nutritious and healthier options. That is one excellent benefit of the ketogenic balance. As a guideline, look over some of the healthier choices as shown throughout the cookbook chapters.

It is essential to understand which fats are dangerous and which ones are good for your health. You must make a balance between the Omega-6s and the Omega-3s. Tuna, trout, shellfish, and salmon are a beneficial choice for the balance of Omega-3.

Convert the Pantry to Keto

Flours used from seeds and nuts are excellent substitutes for regular flour which can include almond flour and milled flax seeds. Macadamias, almonds, and walnuts are also a good choice if eaten in small amounts.

These are some of the items to get your ketogenic lifestyle started:

- Coconut flour
- Quinoa
- Natural nut butter – no sugar
- Sugar-free gelatin
- Unsweetened cocoa powder
- Pickles (limit sweet or bread & butter)
- Yellow mustard
- Sugar-free ketchup
- Stevia or Splenda

Revamp the Spices

Be sure to read spice labels carefully because many of them have hidden sugar. Add some of these spices to your galley:

- Black Pepper
- Sea Salt
- Cinnamon
- Cayenne Pepper
- Chili Powder
- Basil
- Cilantro

Rethink Your Sweetener Choices

Always be on the lookout for the fillers that could cause spikes in your blood sugar with additional carbs that may include dextrose, maltodextrin, or polydextrose. Some sweeteners are preferred over others, so the final word is all yours. Consider these five choices when you start your next shopping list.

Stevia Drops are offered by *Sweet Leaf* and offer delicious flavors including hazelnut, vanilla, English toffee, and chocolate. Enjoy making a satisfying cup of sweetened coffee and drinks. Some individuals think the drops are too bitter. At first, use only three drops to equal one teaspoon of sugar.

Pyure's Organic All-Purpose Blend is considered the best all-around sweetener with less of a bitter after-taste versus a stevia-based product. The blend of stevia and erythritol is an excellent alternative to baking, sweetening desserts, and various cooking needs. The substitution ratio is one teaspoon of sugar for each one-third teaspoon of Pyure. Add slowly and adjust to your taste since you can always add a bit more. If you need powdered sugar, just grind the sweetener in a NutriBullet or high-speed blender until it's very dry.

Swerve Granular Sweetener is also an excellent choice as a blend. It's made from non-digestible carbs sourced from starchy root veggies and select fruits. Give it a try if you who don't like the taste of stevia. Start with ¾ of a teaspoon for every one of sugar. Increase the portion to your liking. Swerve also has its own confectioners/powdered sugar for your baking needs. On the downside, it is more expensive (about twice the price) than other products such as the Pyure. You have to decide if it's worth the difference.

Lakanto's Maple-Flavored Syrup is an excellent choice for pancake syrup since it is monk-fruit and erythritol based. Golden Monk Fruit Sweetener also has a brown sugar choice. The name monk-fruit came from the Buddhist monks over 1,000 years ago and is considered a cooling agent. It may not agree with your digestive system, so use it sparingly if using in baked goods.

Xylitol is at the top of the sugary list. It is excellent for sweetening your teriyaki and BBQ sauce. It tastes just like sugar! The natural occurring sugar alcohol has the Glycemic index (GI) standing of 13. If you have tried others and weren't satisfied, this might be for you.

Xylitol is also known to keep mouth bacteria in check which goes a long way to protect your dental health. The ingredient is commonly found in chewing gum. Unfortunately, if used in large amounts, it can cause diarrhea - making chewing gum a laxative if used in large quantities. *Pet Warning*: If you have a puppy in the house, be sure to use caution since it is toxic to dogs (even small amounts).

Consider the Glycemic Index

Each of these has a GI (Glycemic Index) next to them. This is a measurement of how much your blood sugar is raised after you consume a specific food. If there is a zero (0) next to it; that means it will not increase your blood sugar counts. The measurement can reach 100 which is the baseline of insulin.

- Aspartame – GI: 0
- Erythritol - GI: 0
- Monk Fruit GI: 0
- Xylitol- GI:13
- Sucralose (liquid) GI: Variable
- Stevia (liquid) - GI: 0
- Inulin – GI: 0
- Maltitol – GI:36

- Saccharin – GI: Variable

Recognize Healthy Fats

To achieve success in the ketogenic diet, you need fats. These are some of the healthy fats you will want to keep stocked:

Monounsaturated and Saturated Fats: Avocado, butter, coconut oil, egg yolks, and macadamia nuts are some of the recommended categories. These products can be incorporated into your meals using dressings, sauces, or a bit of butter on your meats.

Use non-hydrogenated lards, coconut oil or ghee. Less oxidation occurs in the oil because they have higher smoke points than other oils. Consider these healthy fat options:

- Avocado oil
- Extra-virgin olive oil (EVOO)
- Coconut Oil
- Sesame oil
- Flaxseed oil
- Olives
- Coconut flakes

Nuts & Seeds: Almonds, Walnuts, Pumpkin seeds, chia seeds, flaxseeds, etc.

Stock the Refrigerator

- Heavy whipping cream

- Sour cream

- Cream cheese

- Goat cheese

- Soft and hard cheeses (for example sharp cheddar, or mozzarella)

- Parmesan cheese

- Kefir

- Grass-Fed Butter: You can promote fat loss and is almost carb-free. The butter is a naturally occurring fatty acid, which is rich in conjugated linoleic acid (CLA). It is suitable for maintaining weight loss and retaining lean muscle mass.

- Ghee – also called clarified butter

- Whole Eggs: Omega-3 eggs, whole eggs, & pasteurized eggs. Visit your local area market for free-range options. You can scramble, fry, boil, or devil eggs up for a picnic or any occasion.

Stock Your Kitchen with Fresh Fruits

- This collection of keto fruits will offer you under 7 grams of net carbs per 1/2 cup or 100 grams:
- Lemon juice
- Lime juice
- Strawberries
- Casaba Melon
- Green olives
- Avocados
- Coconut
- Rhubarb
- Black Olives
- Carambola aka Starfruit
- Gooseberries
- Prickly pears
- Acerola, aka West Indian Cherry
- Oheloberries
- Boysenberries
- Grapefruit

Consider raspberries; many of the professionals believe this is one of the healthiest and most nutritious fruits. A 1/2 cup serving merely carries 5.4 net carbs as well as many health-protective polyphenols which help fight oxidative stress. A handful is enjoyable with a splash of heavy cream.

What about blackberries? This is a delicious 5 net carbs for a 1/2 cup serving. Add some heavy cream.

Stock Up With Healthy Vegetables

Each of these has the Net Carbs listed per 100 grams or 1/2 cup:

- Alfalfa Seeds – Sprouted - 0.2
- Arugula – 2.05
- Asparagus – 1.78
- Bamboo shoots: 3
- Beans – Green snap – 3.6
- Beet greens – 0.63
- Bell pepper
- Broccoli – 4.04
- Broccoli raab – 0.15
- Cabbage – savoy – 3
- Carrots – 6.78
- Carrots – baby – 5.34
- Cauliflower – 2.97

- Celery – 1.37

- Chard – 2.14

- Chicory greens – 0.7

- Chives – 1.85

- Coriander – Cilantro Leaves – 0.87

- Cucumber with Peel – 3.13

- Eggplant – 2.88

- Garlic – 30.96

- Ginger root – 15.77

- Kale – 5.15

- Leeks – bulb (+) lower leaf – 12.35

- Lemongrass – citronella 25.31

- Lettuce – red leaf – 1.36

- Lettuce – crisp-head types ex. iceberg 1.77

- Mushrooms brown – 3.7

- Mustard Greens – 1.47

- Onions – yellow – 7.64

- Onions – scallions or spring – 4.74

- Onions – sweet – 6.65

- Peppers – banana – 1.95

- Peppers – red hot chili – 7.31

- Peppers – jalapeno – 3.7

- Peppers – sweet – green – 2.94

- Peppers – sweet – red – 3.93

- Peppers – sweet – yellow – 5.42

- Portabella Mushrooms – 2.57

- Pumpkin – 6

- Radishes – 1.8

- Seaweed – kelp – 8.27

- Seaweed – spirulina - 2.02

- Shiitake mushrooms – 4.29

- Spinach – 1.43

- Squash 0 crookneck, summer – 2.64

- Squash - Zucchini – 2.11

- Squash – winter – acorn – 8.92

- Tomatoes – 2.69

- Turnips – 4.63

- Turnip Greens – 3.93

- White Mushrooms – 2.26

Special Notes:

- Kale: Your heart health can be significantly improved with the rich nutrients including magnesium and folate.

Build Your Protein Levels
Protein Products

The keto plan focuses on quality proteins, not carbohydrates. You will see many items listed as a starting point.

- Fatty Fish: Tuna: Fresh & Canned - Salmon: Fresh wild caught salmon – portioned in bags to freeze - trout - mackerel,

- Shrimp

- Fresh nuts: Macadamia, sesame seeds, flax seeds, chia seeds, etc.

- Turkey: Breasts & ground turkey

- Chicken: Thighs, breasts, drumsticks, & ground chicken

- Pastured Pork & Poultry: Choose from duck, chicken, pheasant, or quail.

- Beef: Flank steak, chuck roast, sirloin, lean ground beef

- Venison: This is an excellent choice since it is lean, as well as vegetarian-raised meat.

- Peanut Butter: Try natural peanut butter but use caution because they do contain high counts of carbohydrates and Omega-6s. Macadamia nut butter is a wise alternative.

Beverage & Sweetener Options

As always, the number one recommendation for a beverage is water. You can also flavor your drinks using lemon juice or stevia-based flavorings. Consider some of these drink choices. This chart is calculated with your grams of carbs derived for you.

- Water: -0-
- Water with lemon: -0-
- Tea -0- 1 sugar cube = 4 grams
- Coffee -0-
- Diet soft drink -0- Beware of artificial sweeteners
- 8 oz. Almond milk, unsweetened: 2
- 1 cup coconut water: 9
- 1 cup soy milk: 12
- 1 cup orange juice: 26

Enjoy Your Coffee & Tea: If you are struggling during your dieting plan, it is always good to know you can enjoy black coffee and unsweetened tea for -0- net carbs. It is also essential to maintain your health using dairy products. It is best to choose fresh/raw or organic milk products. You can also add additional protein and calcium using non-dairy products such as cashew or almond milk. Try Bulletproof Coffee — it is one of the best keto-friendly drinks!

How to Adjust - High-Carb to Low-Carb Substitutions

As you begin your new and healthier lifestyle, you will discover many shortcuts or substitutes to help you stay on track. Some of these replacements will help:

- **Flour:** Almond flour only contains 3 grams of carbs for 1/4 of a cup. Coconut flour has 6 grams, but totals are overwhelming for the regular wheat flour at 24 grams. This is why it is not on your diet plan!

- **Breadcrumbs**: You can still enjoy your crunchiness by replacing regular breadcrumbs with crushed pork rinds. The good news is that the pork rinds have zero carbs. Next time, enjoy healthier fats.

- **Tortillas**: Get ready to say no to this one which weighs in at approximately 98 grams for just 1 serving. Instead, enjoy a lettuce leaf at about 1 gram per serving. You will still have the 'healthy' crunch!

- **Regular Rice**: Replace the standard serving portions of white or brown rice with some cauliflower rice. You can enjoy 1 cup for about 45 grams of carbs versus the 2.5 grams packed in for 1 cup of its partner.

- **Pasta**: Replace pasta with zucchini. You use a spiralizer and make long ribbons to cover your plate. It is excellent for many dishes served this way.

- **Mashed Potatoes**: Kick the regular bowls of mashed potatoes to the side and enjoy some mashed cauliflower.

Chapter 2

Keto Breakfast & Brunch Specialties

No matter what time the clock chimes; one of these dishes will surely please even the choosiest eater!

ASPARAGUS & BACON MUFFINS

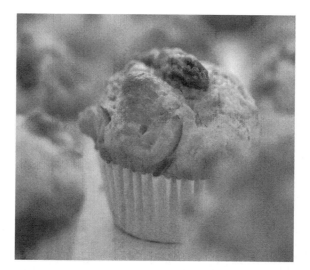

Servings: 12 – 3 muffins each

Macros: 3 g Net Carbs | 41 g Fat | 19 g Protein | 460 Cal.

Ingredients:

- Diced bacon slices – 4 slices
- Whisked eggs - 8
- Asparagus spears - 1 c. chopped or 7-8 pieces
- Chopped onions – 2 tbsp.
- Pepper and salt – to taste
- Coconut milk – canned – .5 cup

Preparation Method:

1. Heat up the oven until it reaches 350°F.

2. Prepare the bacon to your liking and drain on a towel. Dice when cooled.

3. Combine all of the fixings for the muffins and add to 12 mini quiche cups.

4. Bake until the center is set (25 to 30 min.).

AVOCADO & SALMON OMELET WRAP

Servings: 2

Macros: 5.8 g Net Carbs | 67 g Fat | 37 g Protein | 765 Cal.

Ingredients:

- Pepper & Salt – Pinch of each
- Large eggs - 3
- Cream cheese - full-fat – 2 tbsp.
- Freshly chopped chives – 2 tbsp.
- Butter/ghee - 1 tbsp.
- Smoked salmon - .5 pkg. or 1.8 oz.
- Avocado - 3.5 oz. - .5 of an average sized one
- Spring onion - 1

Preparation Method:

1. In a mixing bowl, add a pinch of pepper and salt along with the eggs. Use a fork or whisk - mixing well. Blend in the chives and cream cheese.

2. Prepare the salmon and avocado; peel and slice.

3. In a skillet, add the butter or ghee, and the egg mixture. Cook until fluffy and soft. Put the omelet on a serving dish and spoon the combination of cheese over it.

4. Sprinkle the onion, prepared avocado, and salmon into the wrap. Close and serve.

CINNAMON APPLE SPICED MUFFINS

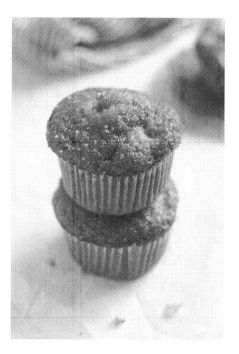

Servings: 12

Macros: 4 g Net Carbs | 17 g Fat | 7 g Protein | 198 Cal.

Ingredients:

- Melted coconut oil or butter – .25 cup

- Super-fine almond flour – 2.5 cups

- Cinnamon - 1 tsp.

- Granulated stevia-erythritol blend – .75 cup

- Baking powder - 1 tsp.

- Sea salt – .5 tsp.

- Large eggs – 4

- Vanilla extract- 1 tsp.

- Almond milk – Unsweetened - .25 cup

- Granny Smith apple – 1 – 4 oz.

Preparation Method:

1. Warm up the oven to 350°F. Add liners to a 12-count muffin tin or spritz with some oil.

2. Whisk the stevia, salt, cinnamon, baking powder, and flour in a mixing container. Fold in the coconut oil or butter to make a crumbly mixture.

3. Mix the milk, extract, and eggs in another container.

4. Combine the fixings. Peel, slice and finely dice the apple, and add to the batter.

5. Fill each of the cups about 3/4 of the way to the top.

6. Bake until it springs back when gently touched (approx. 25-30 min.).

7. Leave the muffins in the baking tin for five to ten minutes. Place them on a wire rack to finish cooling.

8. Enjoy when cooled or set aside for when you want a delicious snack.

COFFEE BREAKFAST PUDDING

Servings: 2

Macros: 11.5 g Net Carbs | 24.5 g Fat | 6.3 g Protein | 347 Cal.

Ingredients:

- Herbal coffee – your choice – 2 tbsp.
- Cacao nibs - .25 cup
- Dried chai seeds - .25 cup
- Undiluted coconut cream - .33 cup
- Sweetener – Swerve – 1 pkg.
- Vanilla extract- 1 tbsp.

Preparation Method:

1. Prepare the coffee with 2 tbsp. of herbal coffee. Cook slowly for 15 minutes until it measures one cup.

2. Strain and combine with the coconut cream, vanilla, and swerve.

3. Stir in the chia seeds and cacao. Store in the fridge for 30 minutes.

4. Serve from the refrigerator. Toss a few more nibs for a taste enrichment or a splash more of coffee.

EGG PORRIDGE

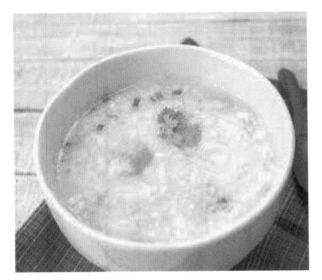

Servings: 1

Macros: 4.7 g Net Carbs | 46.7 g Fat | 12.4 g Protein | 484 Cal.

Ingredients:

- Ground cinnamon - 1 tbsp.

- Eggs - 2

- Heavy cream – .33 cup

- Sugar-free keto-friendly sweetener – 1 packet

- Butter – 2 tbsp.

Preparation Method:

1. Use a small mixing container to whisk the eggs, sweetener, and cream.

2. Heat up a saucepan and melt the butter using the medium-high setting.

3. When melted, lower the temperature, and pour in the egg mixture. Continue to stir until it starts to clump. Take it from the burner.

4. While it's still steaming, enjoy with a dusting of the cinnamon.

HEALTHY HAM MUFFINS

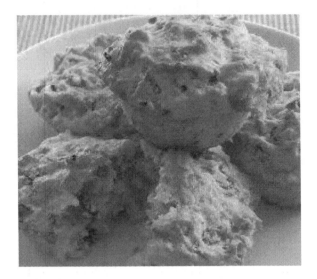

Servings: 12

Macros: 1.5 g Net Carbs | 10 g Protein | 9 g Fat | 129 Cal.

Ingredients:

- Ham – 12 oz.
- Green pepper – .25 cup
- Celery – 1 stalk
- Freshly chopped parsley – 1 tbsp.
- Minced chives – 1 tbsp.
- Pepper – .25 tsp.

- Cayenne – 1 dash

- Onion powder – .25 tsp.

- Shredded cheddar cheese – 6 oz.

- Eggs – 3

Preparation Method:

1. Warm up the oven to 375°F. Line a rimmed baking sheet with foil (for possible spills). Spritz the muffin tins with some cooking spray or oil.

2. Mince the celery and green pepper. Also, finely mince the ham in a food processor. Combine all of the fixings.

3. Spoon into the muffin tins. Bake until browned (30 to 35 min.).

4. Arrange on a cooling rack for about ten minutes. Enjoy piping hot or later as a snack.

KETO CEREAL

Servings: 2

Macros: 5.3 g Net Carbs | 76.8 g Fat | 28.3 g Protein | 1002 Cal.

Ingredients:

- Unsweetened & shredded coconut - .5 cup
- Crushed walnuts - .33 cup
- Salt – 1 dash
- Crushed macadamia nuts - .33 cup
- Butter - 3-4 tsp.
- Flaxseed - 2 cups
- Optional: Sweetener of choice – 2 g. approx.

Preparation Method:

1. Warm up the oven to about 300°F. Toast the nuts and coconut.

2. On the stovetop, warm up a pan using the medium-high temperature setting. Add the butter to melt. Next, just add the nuts and salt. Stir for 2 minutes.

3. Stir in the coconut – continuously stirring. Sprinkle with the milk and sweetener.

4. Let it simmer for one to two minutes. You can also let it soak for ten minutes or enjoy hot.

5. Total time for this treat is only 15 minutes!

PUMPKIN PANCAKES

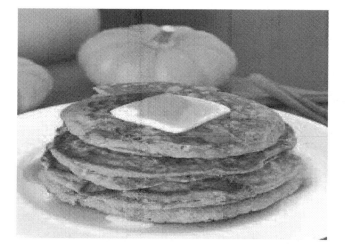

Servings: 6

Macros: 3.3 g Net Carbs | 17.4 g Fat | 5.8 g Protein | 200 Cal.

Ingredients:

- Egg whites – 2 tbsp.
- Eggs - 3

- Ground hazelnuts – 4 tbsp.

- Ground flaxseed – 4 tbsp.

- Baking powder – 1 tsp.

- Coconut cream – 1 cup

- Black tea – ex. Masala Chai – 1 tbsp.

- Vanilla extract – 1 tsp.

- Pumpkin puree - .5 cup

- Sweetener – 5 drops

- Coconut oil – for cooking – 1 tbsp.

Preparation Method:

1. Combine the wet fixings together for about 30 seconds until well mixed.

2. In another dish, whisk the dry fixings.

3. Combine the mixtures well, adding a little of water (up to 1/4 cup) if it's too thick.

4. Add about one teaspoon of the oil to the pan and place on the low-temperature setting.

5. Cover and cook for 2-3 minutes. Flip and continue cooking until done.

6. Serve with a keto-friendly syrup of your liking.

7. Total time is only 35 min.

SPINACH – SAUSAGE & FETA FRITTATA

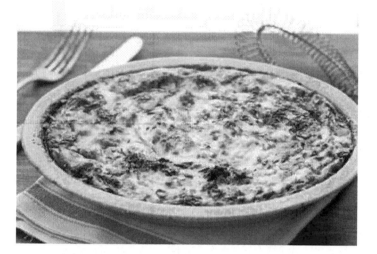

Servings: 9 -2 muffins ea.

Macros: 1.9 g Net Carbs | 24.1 g Fat | 17.3 g Protein | 295 Cal.

Ingredients:

- Sausage – 12 oz.
- Spinach – 10 oz.
- Feta cheese - .5 cup
- Eggs – 12
- Heavy cream - .5 cup
- Salt - .5 tsp.

- Unsweetened almond milk - .5 cup

- Black pepper - .25 tsp

- Ground nutmeg - .25 tsp

- Also Needed: 9x13 baking pan or muffin tins – 18 count

Preparation Method:

1. Warm up the oven temperature to 375°F.

2. Chop the sausage into small bits and place in a mixing bowl.

3. Squeeze dry the spinach and break it apart. Add it in with the sausage.

4. Sprinkle with the feta and gently toss to combine. Add to prepared muffin tins or baking dish. Leave space at the top for the muffin to rise.

5. Bake 50 minutes for the baking pan or 30 minutes for muffins.

6. Enjoy at room temperature or warm.

7. Total time is just 60 minutes for a delicious treat.

TUNA DEVILED EGGS

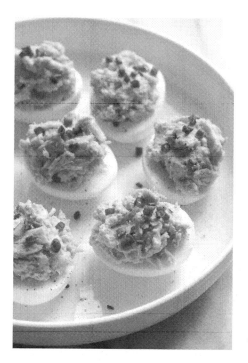

Servings: 4 (4 egg halves ea.)

Macros: 3 g Net Carbs | 16 g Fat | 26.5 g Protein | 264 Cal.

Ingredients:

- Large hard-boiled eggs – 8

- Red wine vinegar – 1 tsp.

- Albacore tuna in water – 2 cans – 6 oz. ea.

- Light mayonnaise – Keto-friendly – .33 cup

- Freshly chopped chives – 2 tsp.

- Minced red onion – 1 tbsp.

- Pepper & Salt – to your liking

Preparation Method:

1. Slice the boiled eggs into halves. Set the white parts aside for now.

2. Combine the mayo and egg yolks. Mash well.

3. Drain the two cans of tuna and add in with the yolks, along with the vinegar, and onions.

4. Prepare the 16 halved eggs and top with a portion of chives to your liking.

WAKE UP BULLETPROOF COFFEE

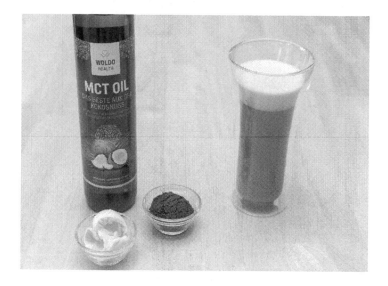

Servings: 1

Macros: -0- g Net Carbs | 51 g Fat | 1 g Protein | 320 Cal.

Ingredients Needed:

- MCT oil powder - 2 tbsp.

- Ghee/butter - 2 tbsp.

- Hot coffee – 1.5 cups

Preparation Method:

1. Pour the hot coffee into your blender.

2. Add the powder and butter. Blend until creamy and frothy.

3. Enjoy served in a large mug at home or on-the-go.

CHAPTER 3

Salad -Veggies - Sides & Supplemental Condiments

These are some tasty luncheon choices or just an extra dish on the side.

BOK CHOY SALAD WITH TOFU

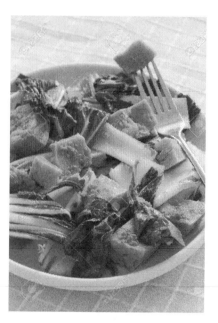

Servings: 3

Macros: 6 g Net Carbs | 36 g Fat | 26 g Protein | 440 Cal.

Ingredients for the Tofu:

- Firm tofu – 15 oz.

- Minced garlic – 2 tsp.

- Red wine vinegar – 1 tbsp.

- Lemon – juiced - .5 of 1

- Sesame oil – 1 tbsp.

- Keto-friendly soy sauce – 1 tbsp.

- Water – 1 tbsp.

Ingredients for the Salad:

- Green onion stalk - 1

- Soy sauce – 2 tbsp.

- Coconut oil – 3 tbsp.

- Sambal Oelek – 1 tbsp.

- Keto-friendly peanut butter – 1 tbsp.

- Chopped cilantro – 2 tbsp.

- Liquid stevia – 7 drops

- Lime -juiced - .5 of 1

- Bok choy – 9 oz.

Preparation Method:

1. Press dry the tofu (6 hrs.) and mix all of the marinade fixings well. Pour into a plastic zipper baggie. Chop the tofu and drop into the marinade. Let it rest overnight in the fridge.

2. Warm up the oven to 350°F. Arrange the tofu on a layer of parchment paper on a baking tin. Bake for 35 minutes.

3. Meanwhile, stir all of the salad fixings except for the Bok choy. Mix well.

4. Once the Bok choy is the size you want, remove the tofu from the oven and enjoy your salad.

5. If you want to enjoy this treat for lunch tomorrow; just prepare it tonight, so it's ready to enjoy by lunchtime.

CAPRESE SKEWERS

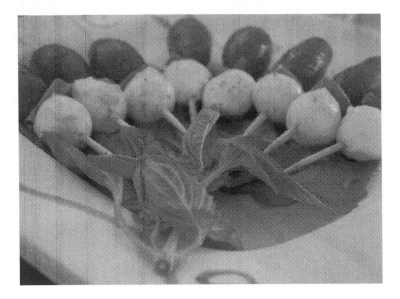

Servings: 2 - 3 skewers each

Macros: 7.1 g Net Carbs | 27.4 g Fat | 24.5 g Protein | 384 Cal.

Ingredients:

- Pitted mixed olives - .5 cup

- Baby mozzarella cheese balls - 2 cups

- Cherry or baby heirloom tomatoes - 2 cups

- Green or red pesto - 2 tbsp.

- Fresh basil - 2 tbsp.

Preparation Method:

1. Rinse the basil and tomatoes. The Kalamata and green olives are delicious when marinated in extra-virgin olive oil and oregano.

2. Combine the mozzarella with the pesto.

3. Arrange the olives, mozzarella, and tomatoes onto the skewers and garnish with the basil.

4. Garnish and let your imagination do the rest.

CARAMELIZED GARLIC MUSHROOMS

Servings: 4

Macros: 2.9 g Net Carbs | 5.2 g Fat | 0.1 g Protein | 75 Cal.

Ingredients:

- Pepper and Salt – to taste
- Butter – 1 tbsp.
- Olive oil – 2 tsp.
- Portobello mushrooms – 1 lb. sliced
- Minced garlic cloves - 2
- Soy sauce – 1 tbsp.

Preparation Method:

1. Add the oil to a skillet using the medium heat setting. Once it's hot, stir in the garlic. Saute until fragrant or about half of a minute or so.

2. Next, add the mushrooms and saute for another 3 minutes. You will see them caramelize.

3. Stir in the salt, pepper, and soy sauce. Saute for 4 additional minutes.

4. Serve and enjoy as a delicious side dish or a treat.

CAULIFLOWER & CHEESE

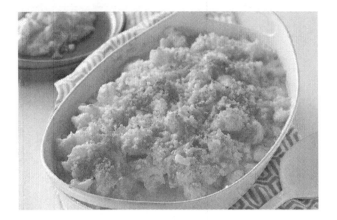

Servings: 4

Macros: 7 g Net Carbs | 23 g Fat | 11 g Protein | 294 Cal.

Ingredients:

- Cauliflower – 1 head

- Cheddar cheese – 1 cup

- Butter – 3 tbsp. - divided

- Heavy cream – .25 cup

- Freshly cracked black pepper & Sea salt – to your liking

- Unsweetened almond milk – .25 cup

Preparation Method:

1. Use a sharp knife to dice the cauliflower into small florets and shred the cheese. Warm up the oven until it reaches 450°F. Cover a cookie sheet with aluminum foil.

2. Melt 2 tablespoons of the butter in a saucepan. Toss the florets and butter together. Dust them with a shake of salt and pepper. Put the cauliflower on the prepared pan and bake for 10-15 minutes.

3. Warm up the rest of the butter, heavy cream, milk, and cheese in a double boiler or microwave.

4. Pour the cheese over the cauliflower and serve.

SUPPLEMENTAL CONDIMENTS

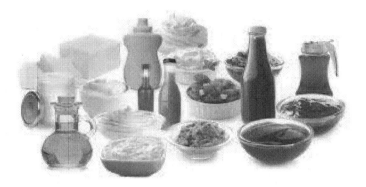

You may be faced with the problem of how to remain in ketosis and still enjoy the condiments that are offered in most supermarkets (you cannot). You are probably wondering how to prepare a keto-friendly meal. If so, this short segment is a special bonus for some of those times when nothing else will work in your favorite keto recipe. These are so delicious that you will not realize, they are very healthy choices.

Keep your ketosis in line with one of these favorites:

AVOCADO MAYONNAISE

Servings: 4

Macros: 4 g Net Carbs | 5 g Fat | 1 g Protein

Ingredients:

- Ground cayenne pepper - .5 tsp.
- Pink salt – 1 pinch
- Lime juice - .5 of 1
- Avocado - .5 of 1 medium
- Olive oil - .25 cup

Preparation Method:

1. Dice the avocado. In a blender or food processor, combine the avocado, salt, cayenne, cilantro, and lime juice.

2. When smooth, stir in the oil – 1 tbsp. at a time - pulsing in between each addition.

3. You can store the mayo for up to one week in a sealed glass bottle.

BLUE CHEESE CHUNKY STYLE DRESSING

Servings: 4

Macros: 3 g Net Carbs | 32 g Fat | 7 g Protein

Ingredients:

- Mayonnaise - .5 cup
- Sour cream - .5 cup
- Lemon juice - .5 of 1
- Worcestershire sauce - .5 tsp.
- Black pepper and salt – to your liking
- Crumbled blue cheese – 2 oz.

Preparation Method:

1. Whisk all of the fixings except for the cheese until well mixed.

2. Fold in the cheese gently and store in a closed glass dish for up to one week.

CAESAR DRESSING

Servings: 4

Macros: 2 g Net Carbs | 23 g Fat | 2 g Protein

Ingredients:

- Mayonnaise - .5 cup
- Dijon mustard – 1 tbsp.
- Lemon juice - .5 of 1
- Worcestershire sauce - .5 tsp.
- Parmesan cheese - .25 cup
- Pinch of each:
- Freshly cracked black pepper – 1 pinch
- Pink Himalayan salt – to taste

Preparation Method:

1. Whisk the lemon juice, mustard, mayonnaise, salt, pepper, and Worcestershire sauce. Stir well and add the parmesan.
2. Whisk until smooth.

3. You can store up to one week in a glass container in the fridge.

SRIRACHA MAYO

Servings: 4

Macros: 2 g Net Carbs | 22 g Fat | 1 g Protein

Ingredients:

- Sriracha sauce – 2 tbsp.
- Paprika - .25 tsp.
- Mayonnaise - .5 cup
- Onion - .5 tsp.
- Garlic - .5 tsp.

Preparation Method:

1. Whisk the fixings together in a small container.
2. Store in an airtight glass container for up to one week in the fridge.

CHAPTER 4

Poultry & Pork Delights

You can mix and match with the delicious chicken, pork, and other combinations in this section!

CHICKEN & BACON PATTIES

Servings: 10 patties

Macros: 1.45 g Net Carbs | 1.45 g Fat| 7.25 g Protein | 95.6 Cal.

Ingredients:

- Bacon - 4 slices
- Chicken breast - 1 can - 12 oz.
- Medium bell peppers - 2
- Large egg - 1
- Sun-dried tomato pesto - .25 cup
- Parmesan cheese - .25 cup
- Coconut flour - 3 tbsp.
- Also Needed: Food processor

Preparation Method:

1. In the food processor, finely chop the peppers and add them to a mixing container. Use a paper towel to remove any of the extra juices.

2. Cook the bacon until crispy. Cool and chop it in with the chicken. Add it to the processor until almost smooth. Combine all of the fixings and make patties.

3. Fry on the medium-high to medium setting in a skillet with a spritz of oil. Once browned on one side, flip it, and continue cooking until done.

4. Drain the grease on paper towels before serving.

5. Garnish with your favorites, but remember to count any extra carbs.

CHICKEN KORMA – INSTANT POT

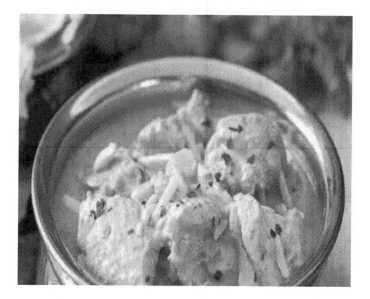

Servings: 6

Macros: 6 g Net Carbs | 19 g Fat | 14 g Protein | 256 Cal.

Ingredients:

- Chicken thighs – 1 lb.

- Chopped onion - 1

- Cashews or almonds -1 oz.

- Garlic cloves - 5

- Green jalapeno - .5 of 1

- Garam masala – 1 tsp.

- Salt – 1 tsp.

- Turmeric – 1 tsp.

- Cayenne pepper - .5 tsp.

- Ground cumin - .5 tsp.

- Ground coriander - .5 tsp.

- Water - use to rinse the blender jar & add to the pot - .5 cup

Ingredients for Finishing:

- Coconut milk – unsweetened - .5 cup

- Garam masala – 1 tsp.

- Chopped cilantro - .25 cup

Preparation Method:

1. Combine the spices and veggies (1st section). Mix everything together except for the cilantro, coconut milk, and chicken. Add the garam masala last. Pour the sauce into the Instant Pot liner.

2. Add the chicken and manually set it on the high-pressure setting for ten minutes. Do a natural pressure release and remove the chicken. Chop it into bite-sized pieces.

3. Pour in the milk and garam masala. Transfer back to the pot to warm.

4. Serve when ready and garnish with cilantro if you like.

CHICKEN SATAY

Yields: 3 Servings

Macros: 3.5 g Net Carbs | 22 g Fat | 34 g Protein | 390 Cal.

Ingredients:

- Ground chicken - 1 lb.
- Chili paste - 2 tsp.
- Sesame oil - 2 tsp.
- Rice vinegar - 1 tbsp.
- Erythritol - 1 tbsp.
- Cayenne pepper - .25 tsp.
- Paprika - .25 tsp.
- Minced garlic - 1 tsp.
- Yellow bell pepper - .33 of 1
- Keto-friendly soy sauce - 4 tbsp.
- Spring onions - 2
- Lime – juiced - .5 of 1
- Peanut butter - 3 tbsp.

Preparation Method:

1. Heat up a skillet using the med-high heat setting and add the oil. When hot, add the chicken. Cook until lightly browned.

2. Fold in the rest of the fixings except for the yellow pepper and onion.

3. When done, stir in the onion and yellow pepper. Continue cooking until the onion is translucent (5 min.). Sprinkle with the pepper and salt and enjoy.

CHICKEN STIR FRY WITH BACON

Servings: 3

Macros: 8 g Net Carbs | 29 g Fat | 36 g Protein | 450 Cal.

Ingredients:

- Broccoli florets – 3 cups
- Spinach – 3 cups
- Salted butter – 2 tbsp.
- Minced garlic – 2 tsp.
- Parmesan cheese - .5 cup
- Tomato sauce - .5 cup
- Red wine - .25 cup
- Black pepper - .5 tsp.
- Salt - .5 tsp.
- Red pepper flakes - .5 tsp.
- Cheddar and bacon chicken sausages – ex. Johnsonville - 4

Preparation Method:

1. Slice the sausage into the desired sizes.

2. Warm up a skillet (high) and add the sausage to brown.

3. Prepare a pot of boiling water. Toss in the broccoli and steam for 5 minutes.

4. Push the sausage to the side, stir in the butter and garlic to saute for one to two minutes.

5. Combine all of the fixings and simmer for 10 minutes. Enjoy!

CREAMY CHICKEN SOUP

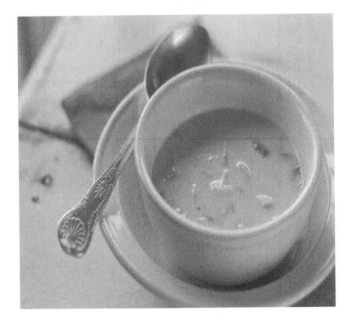

Servings: 4

Macros: 2 g Net Carbs | 25 g Fat| 18 g Protein |307 Cal.

Ingredients:

- Butter - 2 tbsp.

- Breast of chicken 1 large or 2 c. shredded

- Cubed cream cheese - 4 oz.

- Garlic seasoning - 2 tbsp.

- Chicken broth - 14.5 oz.

- Salt - to your liking

- Heavy cream - .25 cup.

Preparation Method:

1. Warm up a saucepan and melt the butter using the medium heat setting.

2. Toss in the shredded chicken. Blend in the cream cheese and seasoning. When melted, add the heavy cream and broth.

3. Once boiling, lower the heat and saute 3-4 minutes. Garnish and season as desired.

KETO "MEATZA" – PIZZA

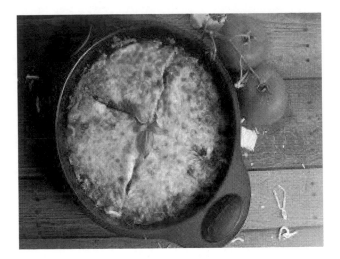

Servings: 2

Macros: 6.75 g Net Carbs | 25.5 g Fat | 46.1 g Protein | 446 Cal.

Ingredients:

- Chicken breast - 12 oz. canned
- Large egg - 1
- Pepper - 1 tsp.
- Basil - 1 tsp.
- Thyme - 1 tsp.
- Garlic - 1 tsp.
- Rosemary - 1 tsp.

- Oregano - .5 tbsp.

- Low-carb tomato sauce - .75 cup

- Mozzarella cheese - 1 cup

- Parmesan cheese - .25 cup

Preparation Method:

1. Warm up the oven temperature to 350°F.

2. Mash the chicken thoroughly in a bowl and add the egg. Sprinkle in the spices and cheese.

3. Add the dough mixture to a pizza pan and crush into the pan with a fork. Toss on the chicken and bake for 15 minutes. It will be done when the edges are browned.

4. Pour on the sauce, add the cheese, and bake for another 15 minutes. Yummy!

LEMON FETA DRUMSTICKS – CROCKPOT

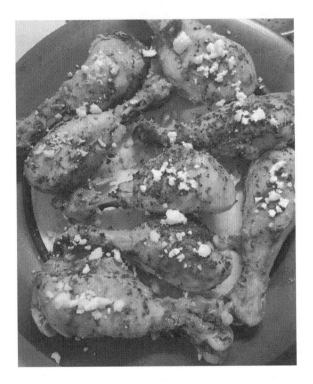

Servings: 4

Macros: 3 g Net Carbs | 7 g Fat | 28 g Protein | 195 Cal.

Ingredients:

- Chicken drumsticks - 8
- Dried oregano – 1 tbsp.
- Grated feta cheese - .33 cup

- Garlic powder – 2 tsp.

- Lemon – juiced - 1

Preparation Method:

1. Remove the skin from the drumsticks. Add each of the fixings into the slow cooker – omitting the feta for now.

2. Cook 4 hours until no longer pink (high setting).

3. When the time's up, sprinkle with the feta and cover. Once the cheese has melted, serve and enjoy.

PORK BELLY & KALE

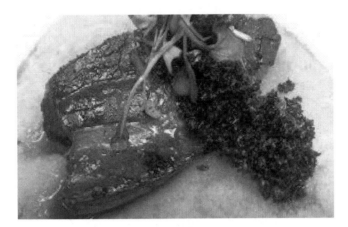

Servings: 4

Macros: 2.3 g Net Carbs | 15.2 g Fat | 3.7 g Protein | 165 Cal.

Ingredients:

- Pork belly - 4 oz.
- Minced garlic clove - 1
- Minced jalapeno - 1
- Apple cider vinegar - 2 tbsp.
- Pink Himalayan salt or Sea salt - to taste

Preparation Method:

1. Prepare the Veggies: Cut the pork into 1/2-inch pieces. Wash and pat dry the kale and discard the hard stems. Shred the leaves. Dice the jalapeno, garlic, and pork.

2. Warm up a cast iron skillet using the med-high heat setting.

3. Brown the pork until crispy (10 min. or so).

4. Toss in the jalapeno and garlic. Saute about 30 seconds.

5. Fold in the kale in batches. When wilted, pour the vinegar into the pan, and simmer until softened (5-10 min.)

6. Store in the refrigerator up to 3 days. Tasty!

7. *Tip*: You can add 2-4 eggs and enjoy for breakfast.

PORK JERK RIBS

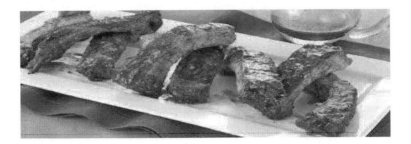

Servings: 6

Macros: 3 g Net Carbs | 20 g Fat | 34g Protein | 320 Cal.

Ingredients:

- Caribbean jerk seasonings - 1 cup
- Baby-back pork ribs – approx. 4 ribs - 1 rack

Ingredients for the Sauce:

- Water - .25 cup
- Tamari/ soy sauce/coconut aminos - .25 cup
- Orange zest - 2 tbsp.
- Chopped fresh ginger - 2 tbsp.
- White vinegar - .25 cup
- Orange juice - .25 cup

- Rice wine vinegar - 2 tbsp.

- Worcestershire sauce - 1 tbsp.

- Dijon mustard - 1 tbsp.

- Arrowroot powder/xanthan gum - 1 tsp.

- Sugar substitute - 3 tbsp.

- Lime Wedges - 2

Preparation Method:

1. Warm up the oven to 375°F.

2. Mix the water, tamari or aminos, mustard, ginger, orange juice, orange zest, white vinegar, rice wine vinegar, and Worcestershire sauce in a small saucepan. Once it boils, simmer for approximately 8 minutes.

3. Strain the sauce to remove the zest and ginger. Add the sauce back into the pan. Mix in the sweetener of choice and xanthan gum until creamy smooth.

4. Thoroughly cover the ribs with the sauce and bake for 30 minutes. Let it rest for ten minutes, slice, and serve. Garnish with a lime wedge or two.

PORK - VEGGIES & NOODLES - INSTANT POT

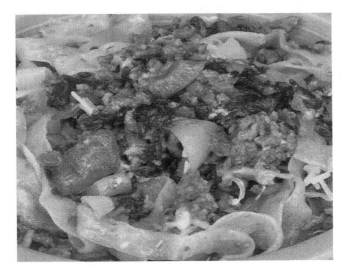

Servings: 6

Macros: 3 g Net Carbs | 18 g Fat | 15 g Protein | 241 Cal.

Ingredients:

- Oil - 1 tbsp.

- Ground pork - 1 lb.

- Chopped bell peppers - 1 cup

- Garlic cloves - 2

- Chopped onion - .5 cup

- Chopped baby spinach - 4 cups

- Shirataki noodles - 2 pkg.
- Grated parmesan cheese - .5 cup

Preparation Method:

1. Use the saute function to warm up the Instant Pot. Add the oil when hot.

2. Toss in the pork and saute until slightly pink. Add the garlic, onions, peppers, and spinach. Scrape the browning bits from the bottom and close the top.

3. Use the high-pressure setting for 3 minutes and quick release the built-up pressure. Pour the sauce over the noodles and garnish with the cheese.

SLOW-COOKED CABBAGE & KALUA PORK

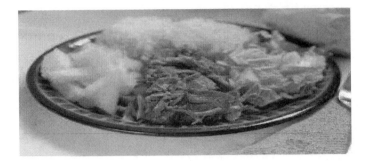

Servings: 12

Macros: 4 g Net Carbs | 13 g Fat | 22g Protein | 227 Cal.

Ingredients:

- Bacon – divided – 7 strips
- Boneless pork shoulder butt roast – 3 lb. approx.
- Head of cabbage - approx. 2 lb. – 1 medium
- Coarse sea salt – 1 tbsp.
- Suggested Size for the Cooker: 6-quarts

Preparation Method:

1. Coarsely chop the cabbage. Trim the fat from the roast.

2. Layer most of the bacon in the cooker. Dust the salt over the roast. Arrange in the cooker over top of the bacon. Place the rest of the bacon on top. Close the lid and cook for 8-10 hours using the low-temperature setting.

3. At that point, toss in the cabbage, and continue cooking covered for one more hour until the cabbage is tender. (It could take a little longer depending on the size of the cooker.)

4. When the roast is done, remove and shred. Use a slotted spoon to arrange the cabbage in the serving dish.

5. Serve with some of the slow cooker juices on the side for dipping. Add your favorite sides.

CHAPTER 5

Beef & Other Favorites

Beef is always a tasty choice if it is cooked just right. Check out some of these delicious meals!

BEEF RIB ROAST FOR SUNDAY

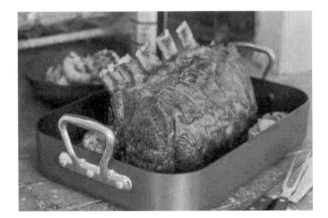

Servings: 8

Macros: 0.5 g Net Carbs |45 g Fat| 92 g Protein | 680 Cal.

Ingredients:

- Black pepper – 1 tsp.
- Sea salt – 2 tsp.

- Garlic powder – 1 tsp.
- Beef rib roast – 5 lb.

Preparation Method:

1. Transfer the roast from the fridge for one hour before time to cook so it can become room temperature. Warm up the oven to 375°F.

2. Rub down the roast with the spices and add to an oven-safe dish or pan. Roast 1 hour.

3. Turn off the oven but *leave the door closed*. Let it rest for 3 hours to make it tender.

4. Transfer the roast to a serving platter. Let it rest for roughly – 15 minutes before slicing.

5. Enjoy any way you like it!

Cheddar-Draped Meatballs

Servings: 24

Macros: 1 g Net Carbs | 8 g Fat | 10 g Protein | 113 Cal.

Ingredients:

- Ground beef – 1.5 lb.
- Chorizo pork sausage – 1.5 lb.
- Chili powder – 1 tsp.
- Cumin – 1 tsp.
- Salt – 1 tsp
- Cheddar cheese – 1 cup
- Large eggs - 2
- Tomato sauce – 1 cup
- Crushed pork rinds - .33 cup

Preparation Method:

1. Warm up the oven until it reaches 350°F. Cover a baking sheet with aluminum foil.

2. Mix the sausage and beef together. Crush the pork rinds and mix in along with the spices, cheese, and eggs.

3. Shape into 24 balls and bake for 35 minutes.

4. When ready to serve, just drizzle with the tomato sauce and enjoy.

Mexican Barbecue

Servings: 9

Macros: 2 g Net Carbs | 11 g Fat | 32 g Prot. | 242 Cal.

Ingredients:

- Chilies in adobo (with the sauce, it's about 4 tsp.) - 2 medium
- Beef or chicken broth - .5 cup
- Chuck roast or beef brisket - 3 lb.
- Minced garlic cloves - 5
- Lime juice - 2 tbsp.
- Apple cider vinegar - 2 tbsp.
- Sea salt - 2 tsp.
- Cumin - 2 tsp.
- Black pepper - 1 tsp.
- Dried oregano - 1 tbsp.
- Whole bay leaves - 2
- Optional: Ground cloves - .5 tsp.

Preparation Method:

1. Mix the chilies in the sauce, and add the broth, garlic, ground cloves, pepper, salt, cumin, lime juice, and vinegar in a blender, mixing until smooth.

2. Chop the beef into 2-inch chunks and toss it in the slow cooker. Empty the puree on top. Toss in the two bay leaves.

3. Cook 4-6 hours on the high setting or 8-10 hours on low. Dispose of the bay leaves when the meat is done.

4. Shred and stir into the juices. Simmer for five to ten minutes.

5. Serve and enjoy.

Steak with Mushroom Port Sauce

Servings: 2

Macros: 6 g Net Carbs | 62 g Fat | 102 g Protein | 984 Cal.

Ingredients:

- Mushrooms – 10 oz.
- Heavy cream – 2 oz.
- Butter – 1 tbsp.
- Port wine – 4 oz.
- Pepper and salt – to taste
- Rib-eye steak – 2 lb.

Preparation Method:

1. Warm up the oven to 450°F. Season the rib-eye steak with pepper and salt.

2. Add the butter to a cast iron skillet on high. Cook the meat for two minutes per side. Add it to a baking pan, cover with foil, and place in the oven.

3. For medium rare, the internal temperature will be 135°F or a total of 12 minutes, flipping halfway through the cooking cycle.

4. Pour the wine into the pan to deglaze. Add the cream and mushrooms and cook until thickened.

5. Serve when it's the way you like it!

STEAK TACOS

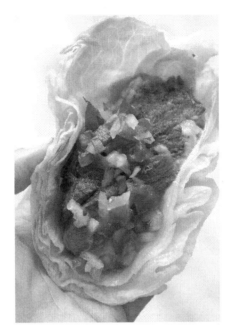

Servings: 4

Macros: 4 g Net Carbs | 8 g Fat | 25 g Protein | 196 Cal.

Ingredients:

- Tri-tip roast – 1 lb.

- Ancho chili powder – 1.5 tsp.

- Salt - .5 tsp.

- Smoked paprika – 1.5 tsp

- Black pepper - .5 tsp.

- Bay leaves – 1-2

- Chopped onion – .5 small

- Garlic cloves - 4

- Beef broth – .5 cup

Preparation Method:

1. Remove the fat from the roast.

2. Smash the garlic into a paste by mincing, using a garlic press or a food processor. Use the back of a knife and some coarse sea salt.

3. Combine the salt, pepper, chili powder, and paprika together to form a rub. Cover the meat.

4. Toss in the onions and empty the beef broth into the slow cooker, adding the meat last. Cook eight hours using the low setting.

5. Remove the lid and shred the meat about 30 minutes from the end of the cycle (7.5 hrs.). Simmer for the last 30 minutes with the lid off.

6. Serve as a lettuce wrap or other favorite choice.

BROILED TILAPIA PARMESAN

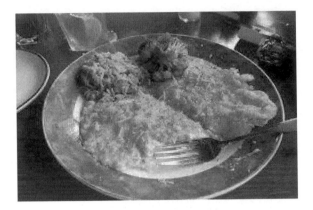

Servings: 8

Macros: 0.8 g Net Carbs | 12.8 g Fat | 25 g Protein | 224 Cal.

Ingredients:

- Melted butter - .25 cup

- Fresh lemon juice - 2 tbsp.

- Parmesan cheese - .5 cup

- Mayonnaise - 3 tbsp.

- Ground black pepper - .25 tsp.

- Dried basil - .25 tsp.

- Celery salt - .125 tsp.

- Onion powder - .125 tsp.

- Tilapia fillets - 2 lb.

Preparation Method:

1. Warm up the oven broiler. Prepare a baking pan with foil or grease it with a spritz of cooking oil spray.

2. Combine the lemon juice, cheese, mayonnaise, and butter in a small dish. Toss in the onion powder, pepper, celery salt, and basil. Stir until mixed. Set aside.

3. Place the tilapia in a pan - single layered. Broil about 2-3 minutes just a few inches from the burners. Flip them over and broil for 2 additional minutes.

4. Take the pan out and sprinkle with the cheese mixture (step 2). Broil about 2 minutes until the fish are flaky. Be careful not to overcook. When the cheese is browned, it should be ready.

GINGER GLAZED SALMON

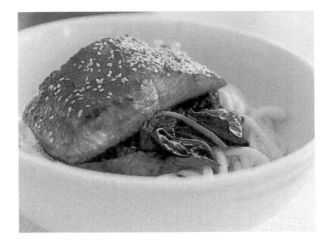

Servings: 2

Macros: 2 g Net Carbs | 22 g Fat | 34 g Protein | 375 Cal.

Ingredients:

- Salmon fillet – 10 oz.
- Minced ginger – 1 tsp.
- Red boat fish sauce – 1 tbsp.
- Rice vinegar – 1 tbsp.
- Sugar-free ketchup – 1 tbsp.
- Minced garlic – 2 tsp.
- Sesame oil – 2 tsp.

- White wine – 2 tbsp.
- Keto-friendly soy sauce – 2 tbsp.

Preparation Method:

1. Combine all of the fixings except for the sesame oil, wine, and ketchup. Marinate for about 15 minutes.

2. Warm up a skillet and add the oil. When hot, arrange the salmon in the oil with the skin-side down.

3. Prepare the fish for 3-4 minutes for each side. Once it's flipped over, stir in all of the marinade fixings. Let it get hot.

4. At that time, transfer the salmon to a platter. Stir in the white wine and ketchup to the juices in the pan.

5. Simmer six minutes. Serve the sauce on the side of the salmon.

LOBSTER SALAD

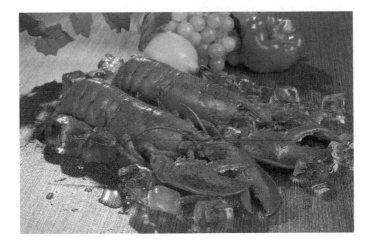

Servings: 4

Macros: 2 g Net Carbs | 25 g Fat | 18 g Protein | 307 Cal.

Ingredients:

- Melted butter - .25 cup
- Keto-friendly Mayonnaise - .25 cup
- Cooked lobster meat – 1 lb.
- Black pepper - .125 tsp.

Preparation Method:

1. Chop the lobster into bite-sized pieces. Melt and pour the butter over the chunks. Toss to coat, and blend in the mayonnaise along with the pepper.

2. Place it into a covered dish for at least ten minutes before serving.

SALMON SALAD

Servings: 4

Macros: 3.5 g Net Carbs | 21.5 g Fat | 26.4 g Protein | 320 Cal.

Ingredients for the Salmon:

- Salmon fillets – 2 - 8 oz. portions
- Freshly cracked ground pepper - pinch
- Himalayan salt – 1 pinch

Ingredients for the Salad:

- Tomato - 1
- English cucumber - .5 of 1
- Green onions - 2
- Celery sticks - 4

Ingredients for the Dressing:

- Garlic clove - 1
- Mustard seeds – 1 tsp.
- Flat leaf parsley - .25 cup

- Black pepper - 1 pinch

- Fresh thyme leaves - 4 bunches - .75 tsp.

- Fresh rosemary leaves - 2 sprigs

- Sea salt - .25 tsp.

- Gluten-free Dijon mustard – 2 tbsp.

- Fresh lemon juice – 2 tbsp.

- Olive oil– 2 tbsp.

- Water

Preparation Method:

1. Slice the cucumber in half lengthwise, then slice. Dice the celery and tomatoes. Also, finely chop the onions. Roughly chop the parsley.

2. Prepare the oven broiler and cover a cookie sheet with aluminum foil.

3. Arrange the salmon on the foil and coat with the pepper and salt. Broil for four to five inches from the heat - based on ten minutes per inch of thickness. Remove when the top has browned.

4. Cool and break apart in a large salad dish. Toss in the onions, cucumber, celery, and tomatoes. Set to the side for now.

5. Combine the dressing fixings in a food processor or blender until creamy. Empty over the salad. Sprinkle with the mustard seeds and freshly chopped parsley.

6. Serve and enjoy on the bed of greens or as a sandwich filling.

7. Note: You need to use extra-virgin olive oil and gluten-free mustard for this one to be perfect.

CHAPTER 6

Snacks & Fat Bombs

BACON WRAPPED JALAPENO POPPERS

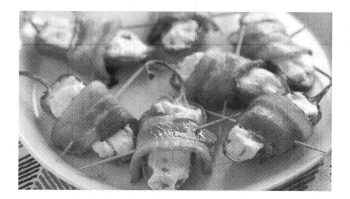

Servings: 4

Macros: 3 g Net Carbs | 18 g Fat | 10 g Protein | 225 Cal.

Ingredients:

- Fresh jalapenos – 16
- Bacon strips - 16
- Cream cheese – 4 oz.
- Paprika – 1 tsp.
- Shredded cheddar cheese - .25 cup

Preparation Method:

1. Warm up the oven until it reaches 350°F. Cover a baking pan with foil.

2. Do the Prep: Cut the ends off of the jalapenos and slice into halves. Discard the seeds. Slice the bacon into 16 pieces.

3. Combine the cream cheese and cheddar. Fill each of the peppers and wrap with the bacon (as in the picture). Arrange on the prepared pan and bake 20-25 minutes.

4. Serve any time for a spicy treat.

CHICKEN LIVER SPREAD

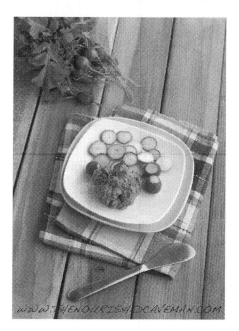

Servings: 1

Macros: 1.5 g Net Carbs | 42.4 g Fat| 24.9 g Protein | 225 Cal.

Ingredients:

- Chicken livers – 3.5 oz.

- Pepper and Salt - 1 pinch or to taste

- Italian seasoning – 1 tsp.

- Softened butter – 3 tbsp.

Preparation Method:

1. Add all of the fixings into a blender to form a paste.

2. Enjoy on radish slices or crackers.

KALE CHIPS

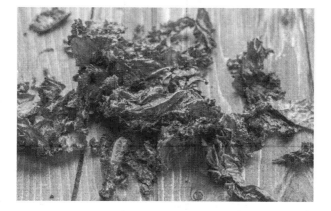

Servings: 2

Macros: 0.5 g Net Carbs | 4 g Protein | 8 g Fat | 180 Cal.

Ingredients:

- Kale - 1 bunch
- Olive oil – 2 tbsp.
- Red pepper – Crushed - 1 tsp.
- Parmesan cheese – 2 tbsp.
- Garlic powder – 1 tsp.

Preparation Method:

1. Warm up the oven until it reaches 350°F.

2. Wash and dry the kale and rip it into pieces (as shown in the picture).

3. Spritz the oil over the kale pieces, add the spices, and gently toss.

4. Evenly arrange the kale on a baking tin. Bake for 8 minutes. If they are not done, continue baking, checking at 2-minute intervals (12 min. should be sufficient.).

5. Cool them down for several minutes and enjoy when they're crunchy the way you like them.

SMOKED BACON FRIES

Servings: 6

Macros: 1.1 g Net Carbs | 31.6 g Fat | 28 g Protein | 409 Cal.

Ingredients:

- Smoked bacon – 1 lb.
- Mustard seeds – 1 tsp.
- Paprika – 1 tbsp.

Preparation Method:

1. Heat up the oven to 360°F.
2. Cut the bacon into small squares and bake for 12-15 minutes.
3. Add the flavorings of paprika and mustard seeds.
4. Enjoy any time!

TOASTED SESAME CRACKERS

Servings: 6

Macros: 3 g Net Carbs | 17 g Fat | 11 g Protein | 213 Cal.

Ingredients:

- Toasted sesame seeds – .25 cup
- Almond flour – 1 cup
- Grated asiago cheese – .5 cup
- Egg white – 1
- Dijon mustard – 1 tbsp.
- Salt – .5 tsp.
- Paprika – 1 tsp.

Preparation Method:

1. Heat up the oven until it reaches 325°F. Lightly grease a baking tin or cover with aluminum foil.

2. Combine all of the fixings except for the salt into a food processor. Pulse until it shapes into dough.

3. Take it from the processor and roll out the dough to form a log (1.5 in. round). Slice them into 1/4-inch slices.

4. Arrange on the baking sheet and sprinkle with the salt.

5. Bake for 17 to 20 minutes.

TURKEY CLUB PINWHEELS

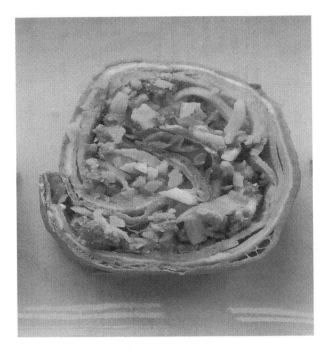

Servings: 3

Macros: 12 g Net Carbs | 36 g Fat | 33 g Protein | 508 Cal.

Ingredients:

- Almond flour tortillas - 4
- Keto-friendly mayonnaise – .25 cup
- Cooked bacon – 4 slices
- Sliced deli turkey – 8 oz.

- Monterey Jack cheese – 4 slices

- Thinly sliced tomato – 1 small

- Chopped lettuce leaves - 2-3

Preparation Method:

1. Prepare the Wraps: Spread the mayo over each of the tortillas. You can also use lettuce as the wrap instead of a tortilla.

2. Layer even portions of turkey, bacon, cheese, tomatoes, and lettuce.

3. Roll into a wrap and slice each one into 6 segments. Serve or refrigerate in a closed dish for up to 4 days.

ANY TIME FAT BOMBS

MEDITERRANEAN FAT BOMBS

Servings: 5

Macros: 1.7 g Net Carbs | 17.1 g Fat | 3.7 g Protein | 164 Cal.

Ingredients:

- Ghee or butter - .25 cup

- Cream cheese - .5 cup

- Pitted olives - 4

- Drained, sun-dried tomatoes (0.4 oz.) 4 pieces

- Crushed garlic cloves - 2

- Pink Himalayan salt - .25 tsp.

- Black pepper –Pinch of freshly ground

- Grated parmesan cheese – 5 tbsp.

- Freshly chopped herbs – 2-3 tbsp. - ex. oregano, basil, and thyme or 2 tsp. dried

Preparation Method:

1. Chop and combine the butter or ghee with the cream cheese after it has softened for about 20 to 30 minutes. Mash it and add the olives and tomatoes.

2. Blend in the pepper, salt, garlic and your choice of dried herbs. Place it in the refrigerator for 20 to 30 minutes until firm.

3. Make five balls with an ice-cream scooper or spoon. Roll them in the grated cheese and add to a plate.

4. Enjoy immediately or store for up to a week in an airtight container.

PIZZA TIME FAT BOMBS

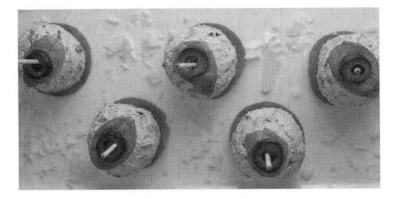

Servings: 6

Macros: 1.3 g Net Carbs | 10.5 g Fat | 2.3 g Protein | 110 Cal.

Ingredients:

- Pepperoni slices - 14

- Cream cheese – 4 oz.

- Pitted black olives - 8

- Fresh chopped basil – 2 tbsp.

- Salt and pepper – to your liking

- Sun-dried tomato pesto – 2 tbsp.

Preparation Method:

1. Chop the olives and pepperoni into small pieces and combine with the remainder of the fixings.

2. Shape the mixture into balls and garnish each one with some pepperoni, olives, and basil.

3. Enjoy any time you need a delicious snack.

WALDORF SALAD - FAT BOMB

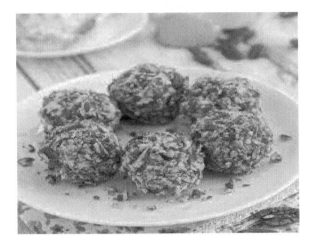

Servings: 6

Macros: 2.5 g Net Carbs | 4.5 g Protein | 19.3 g Fat | 193 Cal.

Ingredients:

- Combine these at room temperature:

- Full-fat cream cheese - 3 oz.

- Unsalted butter or ghee - 2 tbsp.

- Green apple - 2.1 oz. - .5 of a small apple

- Garlic powder - .25 tsp.

- Pepper and salt - to your liking

- Onion powder - .25 tsp.

- Freshly chopped spring onion or chives – 2 tbsp.

- Crumbled blue cheese - .5 cup

- Chopped walnuts or pecans - .66 cup

Preparation Method:

1. Dice the apple into 1/2-inch pieces.

2. Combine the cream cheese and butter in a bowl until smooth. (You can also use a food processor)

3. Fold in the apple, blue cheese, and chives along with the onion and garlic powder. Stir and add the pepper and salt. Place in the fridge for 20 to 30 minutes to set until firm.

4. Scoop out six balls and roll in the chopped nuts of your choice.

5. Enjoy when you wish for up to one week.

CHAPTER 7

Sweet Treats

Take a break with one of the delicious sweets.

BLUEBERRY DELIGHT SMOOTHIE

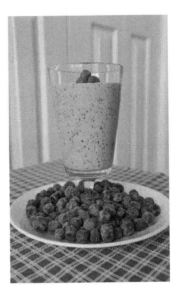

Servings: 1

Macros: 3 g Net Carbs | 21 g Fat | 31 g Protein | 343 Cal.

Ingredients:

- Blueberries - .25 cup
- Coconut milk - 1 cup
- Vanilla essence - 1 tsp.
- MCT oil - 1 tsp.
- Optional: 1 scoop - whey protein powder

Preparation Method:

1. Rinse the blueberries and drain.
2. Toss all of the fixings into a blender.
3. Add a few ice cubes, and blend until creamy smooth.

COCONUT CHIA BARS

Servings: 6 bars

Macros: 3.5 g Net Carbs | 14 g Fat | 4 g Protein | 164 Cal.

Ingredients

- Water - .5 cup
- Chia seeds - 4 tbsp.
- Coconut oil - 1 tbsp.
- Confectioners Swerve - 1 tbsp.
- Vanilla extract - .25 tsp.
- Shredded dried coconut meat - unsweetened - 1 cup
- Cashews - .5 cup
- Also Needed: 9x9 baking sheet

Preparation Method:

1. Set the oven temperature to 350°F.

2. Soak the seeds 15 minutes until gel-like, and mix with the coconut, oil, swerve, and vanilla extract. Lastly, add the cashews.

3. Line the mixture, using parchment paper, on the cookie sheet. Press until it is about a 3/4-inch thickness, and bake for 45 minutes.

4. Slice into six bars and enjoy!

GINGER SNAP COOKIES

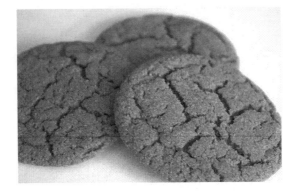

Servings: 1

Macros: 2.2 g Net Carbs | 6.7 g Fat | 2.25 g Protein | 74 Cal.

Ingredients:

- Unsalted butter - .25 cup
- Large egg - 1
- Almond flour - 2 cups
- Ground cinnamon - .5 tsp.
- Vanilla extract - 1 tsp.
- Ground cloves - .25 tsp.
- Nutmeg - .25 tsp.
- Salt - .25 tsp.

Preparation Method:

1. Warm up the oven temperature to 350°F.

2. Whisk the dry fixings in a mixing container. Blend in the remainder of the ingredients into the dry mixture using a hand blender. (The dough will be stiff.)

3. Measure out the dough for each cookie and flatten with a fork or your fingers. Bake for approximately 9-11 minutes or until browned.

LEMON MOUSSE CHEESECAKE

Servings: 1

Macros: 1.7 g Net Carbs | 29.6 g Fat | 3.7 g Prot. | 277 Cal.

Ingredients:

- Lemon juice - 2 lemons approx. - .25 cup
- Heavy cream - 1 cup
- Salt - .125 tsp.
- Cream cheese - 8 oz.
- Lemon liquid stevia - 1 tsp.

Preparation Method:

1. In a stand mixer, combine the lemon juice and cream cheese until smooth.

2. Add the remainder of the ingredients and whip until blended.

3. Adjust the flavor with sweetener if desired. Place in a serving dish and sprinkle with some lemon zest.

4. Refrigerate until you are ready to enjoy.

PEANUT BUTTER SMOOTHIE

Servings: 1

Macros: 11.1 g Net Carbs | 32.8g Fat | 31 g Protein | 446 Cal.

Ingredients:

- Water – 1 cup
- Heavy cream – .33 cup
- Chocolate whey powder - 1 scoop
- Ice cubes – 2 to 3
- Peanut butter – 1 tbsp.

Preparation Method:

1. Combine all of the fixings in your blender.
2. Pulse until smooth.
3. Enjoy served in a chilled glass

PUMPKIN BARS WITH CREAM CHEESE FROSTING

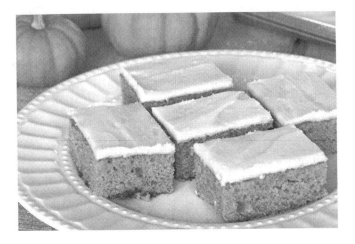

Servings: 16

Macros: 2 g Net Carbs | 13 g Fat | 3 g Protein | 139 Cal.

- Ingredients:
- Large eggs – 2
- Coconut oil – .25 cup
- Pumpkin puree – 1 cup
- Cream cheese – 2 oz.
- Almond flour – 1 cup
- Vanilla extract – 1 tsp.
- Erythritol sweetener blend - .66 cups
- Pumpkin pie spice – 1 tsp.

- Gluten-free baking powder – 2 tsp.
- Sea salt - .5 tsp.

Ingredients for the Frosting:

- Powdered erythritol - .5 cup
- Vanilla extract - 1 tsp.
- Softened cream cheese – 6 oz.
- Optional: Heavy cream – 1 tbsp.
- Also Needed: 9x9 baking pan

Preparation Method:

1. Warm up the oven until it reaches 350°F. Line the baking pan with parchment paper.

2. In a double boiler or microwave, melt the coconut oil, puree, and cream cheese.

3. Mix the vanilla, eggs, cream cheese, and puree using a hand mixer until smooth (medium-speed).

4. Whisk the dry fixings (salt, pie spice, baking powder, sweetener, and flour).

5. Mix all the ingredients with the mixer until just combined and scrape into the pan. Bake for 20 to 30 minutes. Cool completely.

6. Prepare the frosting with each of the ingredients when the bars are cooled. If it's too thick, just add a little cream or milk. Slice into 16 equal portions. Enjoy any time.

CHAPTER 8

14-Day Diet Meal Plan

Please note: Each of the menu items listed in your meal plan is for the grams of net carbs per serving. You can switch the menu to suit your needs since this is set us using the lowest scale of 20 daily grams of carbs. You can add your favorites without guilt!

Day 1:

- Breakfast: Asparagus & Bacon Muffins: 3 g
- Lunch: Bok Choy Salad with Tofu: 0.8 g
- Dinner: Pork Jerk Ribs: 3 g
- Smoked Bacon Fries: 1.1 g
- Snack or Dessert: Blueberry Delight Smoothie: 3 g

Day 1 Totals: 10.9 Net Carbs

Day 2:

- Breakfast: Cinnamon Apple Spiced Muffins: 4 g
- Lunch: Caprese Skewers - 7.1 g
- Toasted Sesame Crackers: 3 g

- Dinner: Broiled Tilapia Parmesan: 0.8 g

- Caramelized Garlic Mushrooms: 3.3 g

- Snack or Dessert: Waldorf Salad - Fat Bomb: 2.5 g

Day 2 Totals: 20.7 Net Carbs

Day 3:

- Breakfast: Keto Cereal: 5.3 g

- Lunch: Lobster Salad: 2 g

- Toasted Sesame Crackers: 3 g

- Dinner: Lobster Salad: 2 g

- Dinner: Chicken Satay: 3.5 g

- Snack or Dessert: Ginger Snaps: 2.2 g

Day 3 Totals: 18 Net Carbs

Day 4:

- Breakfast: Egg Porridge: 4.7 g

- Lunch: Salmon Salad: 3.5 g

- Dinner: Chicken & Bacon Patties: 1.45 g

- Salmon Salad: 3.5 g

- Snack or Dessert: Lemon Mousse Cheesecake: 1.7 g

Day 4 Totals: 14.85 Net Carbs

Day 5:

- Breakfast: Avocado & Salmon Omelet Wrap: 5.8 g
- Lunch: Creamy Chicken Soup: 2 g
- Dinner: Ginger Glazed Salmon: 2 g
- Cauliflower & Cheese: 7 g Net Carbs
- Snack or Dessert: Lemon Mousse Cheesecake: 1.7 g

Day 5 Totals: 18.5 Net Carbs

Day 6:

- Breakfast: Coffee Breakfast Pudding: 11.5 g Net Carbs
- Lunch: Pork - Veggies & Noodles - Instant Pot: 3 g
- Dinner: Beef Rib Roast for Sunday: 0.5 g
- Caramelized Garlic Mushrooms: 3.3 Net Carbs
- Snack or Dessert: Pumpkin Bars with Cream Cheese Frosting: 2 g Net Carbs

Day 6 Totals: 20.3 Net Carbs

Day 7:

- Breakfast: Healthy Ham Muffins: 1.5 g Net Carbs
- Lunch: Mexican Barbecue: 2 g
- Bacon Wrapped Jalapeno Poppers: 3 g
- Dinner: Chicken Stir Fry with Bacon: 8 g
- Snack or Dessert: Coconut Chia Bars: 3.5 g.

Day 7 Totals: 18 Net Carbs

Day 8:

- Breakfast: Pumpkin Pancakes: 3.3 g
- Lunch: Chicken Stir Fry with Bacon: 8 g
- Kale Chips: 0.5 g
- Dinner: Pork Belly & Kale: 2.3 g
- Snack or Dessert: Mediterranean Fat Bombs: 1.7 g

Day 8 Totals: 15.8 Net Carbs

Day 9:

- Breakfast: Tuna Deviled Eggs: 3 g
- Lunch: Keto "Meatza" – Pizza: 6.75 g
- Dinner: Lemon Feta Drumsticks - Crockpot: 3 g
- Snack or Dessert: Pumpkin Bars with Cream Cheese Frosting: 2 g

Day 9 Totals: 14.75 Net Carbs

Day 10:

- Breakfast: Spinach – Sausage & Feta Frittata: 1.9 g
- Lunch: Bok Choy Salad with Tofu: 0.8 g
- Dinner: Slow Cooked Cabbage & Kalua Pork: 4 g
- Snack or Dessert: Peanut Butter Smoothie: 11.1 g

Day 10 Totals: 17.8 Net Carbs

Day 11:

- Breakfast: Asparagus & Bacon Muffins: 3 g
- Lunch: Steak Tacos: 4 g

- Dinner: Turkey Club Pinwheels: 12 g
- Snack or Dessert: Lemon Mousse Cheesecake: 1.7 g

Day 11 Totals: 20.7 Net Carbs

Day 12:

- Breakfast: Cinnamon Apple Spiced Muffins: 4 g
- Lunch: Chicken Korma: 6 g
- Dinner: Lemon Feta Drumsticks - Crockpot: 3 g
- Cauliflower & Cheese: 7 g
- Snack or Dessert: Pizza Time Fat Bombs: 1.3 g

Day 12 Totals: 21.3 Net Carbs

Day 13:

- Breakfast: Healthy Ham Muffins: 1.5 g
- Lunch: Cheddar Draped Meatballs: 1 g
- Dinner: Steak with Mushroom Port Sauce: 6 g
- Cauliflower & Cheese: 7 g Net Carbs
- Snack or Dessert: Bacon Wrapped Jalapeno Poppers: 3g

Day 13 Totals: 18.5 Net Carbs

Day 14:

- Breakfast: Pumpkin Pancakes: 3.3 g
- Lunch: Pork - Veggies & Noodles - Instant Pot: 3 g
- Dinner: Beef Rib Roast for Sunday: 0.5 g
- Snack or Dessert: Peanut Butter Smoothie: 11.1 g

Day 14 Totals: 17.9 Net Carbs

Know What You Are Craving

Now that you have the meal plan; "Do you know what our body is craving?"

As you live a harried lifestyle, sometimes; you just don't know you want. Your body will tell you what is necessary to keep it going. The message is sent to you as a craving. Here are a few 'cravings' with what your body needs and a quick fix for the issue:

- Salty Foods: Your body is craving silicon. So, go grab a few nuts and seeds; just be sure to count them into your daily counts.

- Carbs/Bread/Pasta: You need some nitrogen which can be remedied with some high protein meat.

- Chocolate: The carbon, magnesium, and chromium levels are screaming for some spinach, nuts, and seeds, or some broccoli and cheese.

- Fatty or Oily Foods: The levels of calcium and chloride may need repair. Enjoy some spinach, broccoli, cheese, or fish.

- Sugary Foods: Several things can trigger the desire for sugar, but typically phosphorous, and tryptophan are the culprits. Have some chicken, beef, lamb, liver, cheese, cauliflower, or broccoli.

You may be asking, "What will I do if I am not at home and need to have a quick snack?" You know the feeling, but don't worry, there are choices here too. Remember, the plan is flexible.

Healthy Snacks If You Are On-The-Go

Most convenience stores have just what you need. Choose from one of these snacks:

- Beef Jerky: Watch out for the added sugars if you purchase jerky ready-made. Choose ones with only a few additional ingredients. If you enjoy preparing food, why not try making your homemade jerky. You will know for sure it's healthy!

- Pepperoni Slices: Enjoy with a high-fat cheese but keep in mind, these are highly processed. Limit the amounts used and search for hormone-free or organic if possible.

- Pork Rinds: Use these to replace chips and crackers which are a higher quality without a lot of offensive oil content. For example, try some Parmesan & Pork Rind Green Beans (see the recipe). You can also enjoy 1 14.2 gram serving of pork rinds for -0- net carbs. How does that sound?

- A Slice of Cheese: Enjoy a slice of cheddar cheese, gouda, feta, or some parmesan. However, always check the specific type for the carbohydrate counts.

- String Cheese: Choose the full-fat version without additional fillers.

- Laughing Cow Cheese Wheels: Purchase full-fat versions and get *real* cheese when possible.

- Moon Cheese: Yes, this is real and is a crunchy cheese. It is 100% natural cheese which is similar to potato chips in cheese form.

- Cacao Nibs: You can enjoy the same crunch when used as an alternative to chocolate chips.

- Low-Carb Ice Cream: Breyers CarbSmart gives you the opportunity to enjoy a 1/2 cup portion for only 4 net carbs. It is sweetened with erythritol.

- Greek Yogurt: The fat content is a plus for your ketogenic meal planning. Just be sure you purchase one that has no sugar added. Check each brand for the macros because each one varies. However, it is very filling, and so many are packaged in convenient smaller traveling sizes.

Think Ahead - Prepare Quick Snacks

These are just a few ways always to be prepared for your active life. Take one or two nights each week to make some of these goodies:

- Avocados: This super whole food is a fantastic choice for on-the-go. Slice it into the desired portions (count the carbs) and give it a shake of pepper and salt. Try a sprinkle of grated parmesan for a taste change. You can load up on potassium and magnesium for 1.8 grams of net carbs for a 1/2 cup serving.

- Eggs: Take a few extra minutes to prepare a batch of eggs. Prepared eggs generally store for up to a week in the fridge. It only has 0.9 grams of net carbs per egg. It will also provide you will essential selenium, vitamin A, phosphorus, and folate.

- Cucumbers: Enjoy a crispy cucumber with or without the peel. Enjoy knowing that it is an excellent source of dietary fiber as well as vitamin C and K. Enjoy 1/2 of a cup for only 1 gram of net carbs.

- Cherry Tomatoes: This is an excellent 'handful' treat but one that must be used in small amounts because the carbs do add up quickly. They reel in 2.7 carbs for a 1/2 cup portion. However, they are also a super boost of potassium, vitamin K, biotin, and vitamin C.

- Iced Coffee: Leave the sugar out of your coffee and use only full-fat milk or cream. Add a bit of MCT oil powder, which can be purchased as chocolate, vanilla, or unflavored.

- Olives: Watch out for additional oils added, but this is one great treat right out of the jar.

- Pickles: It is a great day when you can grab a delicious pickle. It is loaded with potassium and sodium to replenish your electrolytes. You can also drink the juice. For a 1-cup portion – it only contains only 1.6 net carbs.

- Nuts & Seeds: Create some tasty meals (in moderation) when adding seeds and nuts to your keto diet plan. Use fattier nuts including macadamias, Brazil nuts, walnuts, and almonds or seeds like chia, pumpkin, and flaxseed, which are high in omega-3's. Use caution and stay away from butter that contains polyunsaturated oils/vegetable oil.

Make a mental note concerning the macadamias; they are high in a heart-healthy fat in olive oil called oleic acid. The macadamia nut has a crunchy taste but on the inside, they're soft.

Conclusion

I am thrilled you have chosen of the *Keto Diet Meal Plan for Beginners: 14-Day Keto Diet Meal Plan for Weight Loss and Healthy Living* as your guideline through ketosis. I hope it was informative and provided you with tons of useful information to help change the rest of your life through each segment of your journey by providing you with the fundamentals of the ketogenic way of living. Each tasty recipe is designed to keep you in ketosis. The first few weeks may be a little stressful but hang in there because it will become easier.

Once you have all of the chief spices and other fixings stocked in your keto kitchen, the following week's shopping list will be much simpler. As a quick reminder, keep these simple tips in mind as you go through your ketogenic journey:

- Drink plenty of water daily and limit the intake of sugar-sweetened beverages.
- It is essential to attempt to use only half of your typical serving of salad dressing or butter.
- Use only fat-free or low-fat condiments.
- Add a serving of vegetables to your dinner and lunch menus.

- Add a serving of fruit as a snack or enjoy with your meal. The skin also contains additional nutrients. Dried and canned fruits are quick and easy to use. However, make sure they don't have added sugar.

- Read the food labels and make choices that keep you in line with ketosis.

- For a snack have some frozen yogurt (fat-free or low-fat), nuts or unsalted pretzels, raw veggies, unsalted-plain popcorn.

- Prepare cut veggies such as bell pepper strips, mixed greens, and carrots. Store them in small baggies for a quick on-the-go healthy choice.

One of the easiest ways to stay on your plan is to remove the temptations. Remove the chocolate, candy, bread, pasta, rice, and sugary sodas you have supplied in your kitchen. If you live alone, this is an easy task. It is a bit more challenging if you have a family. The diet will also be useful for them if you plan your meals using the recipes included in this book.

If you cheat, that has to count also. It will be a reminder of your indulgence, but it will help keep you in line. Others may believe you are obsessed with the plan, but it is your health and wellbeing that you are improving.

When you go shopping for your ketogenic essentials be sure you take your new skills, a grocery list, and search the labels. Almost every food item in today's grocery store has a nutrition label. Be sure you read each of the ingredients to discover any hiding carbs to keep your ketosis in line. You will be glad you took the extra time.

If you have a moment, a comment or two about its contents on Amazon will be much appreciated.

Enjoy your new way of living!

Recipe Index

Pork

- Pork Belly & Kale
- Pork Jerk Ribs
- Pork - Veggies & Noodles - Instant Pot
- Slow Cooked Cabbage & Kalua Pork

Chapter 5: Beef & Other Favorites

1. Beef Rib Roast for Sunday
2. Cheddar Draped Meatballs
3. Mexican Barbecue
4. Steak with Mushroom Port Sauce
5. Steak Tacos

Seafood & Salad

1. Broiled Tilapia Parmesan
2. Ginger Glazed Salmon
3. Lobster Salad
4. Salmon Salad

Chapter 6: Snacks & Fat Bombs

1. Bacon Wrapped Jalapeno Poppers

Any Time Fat Bombs

Chapter 7: Sweet Treats

Made in the USA
San Bernardino, CA
12 May 2019